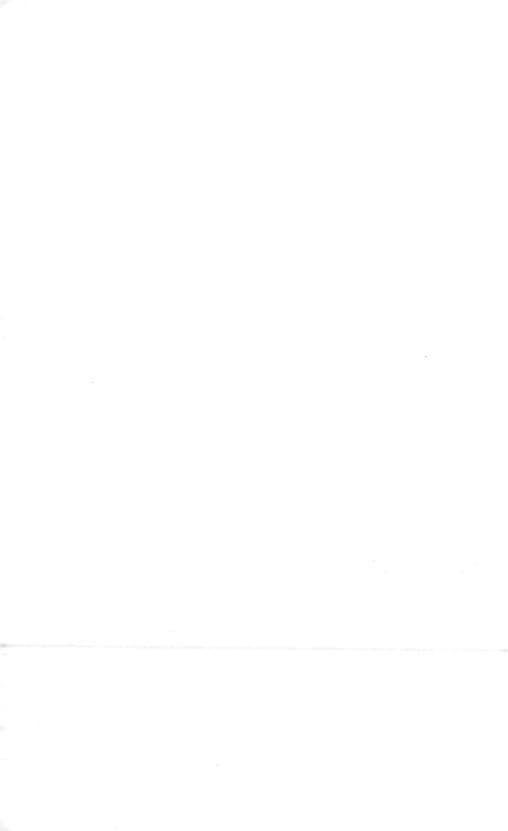

PREVENTIVE MEDICINE
USA

The John E. Fogarty International Center for Advanced Study in the Health Sciences

The Fogarty International Center was established in 1968 as a memorial to the late Congressman John E. Fogarty of Rhode Island. It had been Mr. Fogarty's desire to create within the National Institutes of Health a center for research in biology and medicine, dedicated to international cooperation and collaboration in the interest of the health of mankind. The Fogarty Center is a unique resource within the Federal establishment, providing a base for expanding of America's health research and health care to lands abroad and for bringing the talents and resources of other nations to bear upon the many and varied health problems of the United States.

As an institution for advanced study, the Center has embraced the major themes of medical education, environmental and societal factors influencing health, geographic health studies, preventive medicine, and biomedical research. The Center provides the opportunity for study and discussion of current issues in these and other fields by convening conferences and workshops which bring together U.S. and foreign scientists. In addition, the Center promotes the research of U.S. nationals at institutions abroad and the education and training of foreign scientists in the U.S. through a program of fellowships, scholarships, and study grants.

The American College of Preventive Medicine

The American College of Preventive Medicine is a professional society comprising physicians who are Board certified and/or engaged full time in preventive or community medicine. The membership includes individuals of scientific eminence in practice, teaching, or research in the specialty.

The College promotes continuing medical education and fosters interchange of knowledge and ideas among professionals in preventive medicine through annual meetings, conferences, publications, and joint activities with kindred professional societies.

The society was founded in 1954, six years after the establishment of the American Board of Preventive Medicine, the certifying specialty Board for physicians in the four preventive medicine subspecialties (Public Health, Aerospace Medicine, Occupational Medicine, and General Preventive Medicine).

As the only professional society whose membership encompasses all four subspecialties, the College provides a unique forum for physicians in preventive medicine to speak with one voice from an authoritative position to members of the government and organized medicine.

PREVENTIVE MEDICINE USA

Theory, Practice and Application
of Prevention
in Personal Health Services

Quality Control and Evaluation
of Preventive Health Services

Task Force Reports sponsored by

The John E. Fogarty International Center
for Advanced Study in the Health Sciences
National Institutes of Health

and

The American College of Preventive Medicine

PRODIST
New York
1976

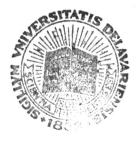

The opinions expressed in this book
are those of the respective authors and
do not necessarily represent those of the
Department of Health, Education, and Welfare.

Library of Congress Catalog Card Number 76-15083
International Standard Book Number 0-88202-105-2

PRODIST

a division of

Neale Watson Academic Publications, Inc.

156 Fifth Avenue, New York, New York 10010

Designed and manufactured in the U.S.A.

Contents

Preface

Theory, Practice and Application of Prevention in
    Personal Health Services

Task Force Members   1

  I   Introduction   2

  II   Rationale   8
      Changing Nature of Health Problems   8
      Empirical Basis for Preventive Medicine   11
      Theoretical Basis for Preventive Medicine   15
      Dynamic Nature of Preventive Medicine   16

  III   Application   18
      History   18
      Factors Influencing Expansion of Preventive
          Medicine   19
      Current Extent of Application   21
      Principles of Application   24

  IV   Issues   27
      Orientation Toward Conditions   27
      Evaluation Criteria   27
      Assessment of Selected Preventive Medicine
          Procedures   30
      Identification of Conditions and Procedures   36
      Justification of Concerted Effort   48
      Implementation of Preventive Medicine   53
      Organization and Financing   56
      Research   58

  V   Conclusions and Recommendations   63

References   64

Appendices   80

Quality Control and Evaluation
    of Preventive Health Services

Task Force Members   103

  I   Introduction   104

  II   Evaluation Methodologies   108
      Penetration Rate   108
      Cost Efficiency   110
      Structure and Organization   111
      Clinical Modalities   112

Laboratory Modalities   129
Health Education Modalities   132
Program Results   139

Summary   143

Recommendations   145

Evaluation Study Examples   149
Family Planning Programs   149
Dental Programs for Children   151
Breast Cancer Screening Programs   153
Early Periodic Screening, Diagnosis, and
Treatment (EPSDT)—Medicaid   155

References   157

Preface

Improvement in the health status of the American people will depend, in great measure, on the design and application of programs which place major emphasis on the preventive aspects of human disease. The nature of our health problems dictates that application of known methodologies in prevention and health maintenance can cause a substantial improvement in our nation's health statistics. Although health authorities generally agree with this thesis, there is need for more precise definition of effective methods and programs of prevention, financial and manpower resources required to implement these programs, and priorities to be assigned to research in preventive methodology.

Leaders throughout the health field, in government, the academic sector, and industry, have expressed repeatedly the need to assemble expertise in order to elucidate mechanisms whereby the full impact of preventive medicine can be brought to bear on the solution of America's major health problems. The Department of Health, Education, and Welfare has evidenced its commitment to prevention in a variety of ways, the most notable being that prevention has been selected as one of the five major themes for development in Departmental programs, as detailed in *The Forward Plan for Health, 1976-1980*. As stated there, "the major element of a preventive strategy is to assure the concentration of all federally supported health programs in preventive health services, health maintenance, and health education." The Department has pledged a full commitment to review of current practice, evaluation of preventive methodology, and the generation of new knowledge.

The Fogarty International Center of the National Institutes of Health, in anticipation of this new emphasis, initiated in 1973 an analysis of preventive medicine. Comprehensive studies were designed to review and evaluate the state-of-the-art of prevention and control of human diseases, to identify deficiencies in knowledge requiring further research, and to recognize problems in application of preventive methods and suggest corrective action. In an effort to contribute to the educational aspects of preventive medicine, the Fogarty Center undertook a cooperative program with the Association of Teachers of Preventive Medicine to conduct workshops and create resource material to assist in the administration, teaching, research, and service responsibilities of departments of preventive medicine, to enhance collaborative activities between these departments and other units of health science schools, and to promote national programs of teaching, research, and service in preventive medicine.

These efforts in preventive medicine, and the close collaboration with experts in this and allied fields, led the Fogarty Center and the American

College of Preventive Medicine to create and support the work of eight Task Forces addressing various components of the field of disease prevention, whose charge was to develop guidelines for a national effort in preventive medicine. The output was to be specifics; that is, concrete proposals whose orientations were pragmatic, programmatic, and realistic. Over 300 specialists participated in preparing these documents with the endorsement and support of health organizations and professional societies with preventive medicine orientations. In June, 1975, the eight reports were presented at the National Conference on Preventive Medicine convened at the National Institutes of Health. The major purposes of the conference were to focus attention on the significant accomplishments of preventive strategies that had been applied to the health problems of this country in recent years and to offer expert opinion on where preventive measures could be expected to yield equally significant health advances in the future. At this meeting, the reports were analyzed during workshop sessions, and their recommendations were discussed and revised until a scientific consensus was reached. The present volume is the culmination of this concerned, long-term effort.

The eight Task Force reports were used as the basis for the Prevention theme of the DHEW *Forward Plan for Health, 1976-1980*, and the recommendations of the reports are being considered by DHEW agency heads for appropriate implementation in their programs. While the debate will continue as to the precise Federal role in developing and executing a national health plan, most observers recognize the paramount position of the Congress and the Executive branch in formulating guidelines for system reform. We anticipate that the documents of the National Conference on Preventive Medicine will provide a base of knowledge on the theory and application of preventive medicine from which national programs might arise.

Milo D. Leavitt, Jr., M.D.
Director
Fogarty International Center

Irving Tabershaw, M.D.
President
American College of Preventive Medicine

Task Force Members

Lester Breslow, M.D., M.P.H., *Chairman*
School of Public Health
University of California, Los Angeles
Los Angeles, California

Robert Haggerty, M.D.
Center for Advance Study in
   The Behavioral Sciences
Stanford University
Stanford, California

Maureen Henderson, M.D.
School of Medicine
University of Maryland
Baltimore, Maryland

Peter Peacock, M.D.
American Health Foundation
New York, New York

Ernest Saward, M.D.
School of Medicine and Dentistry
The University of Rochester
Rochester, New York

Sam Shapiro
Health Services Research
   and Development Center
The Johns Hopkins University
Baltimore, Maryland

Leon Ellwein, PH.D. (Consultant)
Science Applications, Inc.
La Jolla, California

1

I. Introduction

This report reviews the rationale for application of current knowledge in preventive medicine, experience with that application, and issues in the field. The key recommendation is to make available to people a set of packages of preventive medical services, each specific to a particular age-sex group. Rather than a "general, annual check-up," every person would be offered at certain critical periods of life an appropriate package of preventive medical services. These periods of life include pregnancy, infancy, school entry, puberty, entry to adult life, every five years during early and middle adult life, and every two years during later adult life. Each package of preventive medical services includes certain physical procedures, for example, blood pressure determination; and certain counseling procedures, for example, advice pertaining to food and alcohol. The package for each age-period of life comprises specific physical and counseling procedures deemed useful in preserving health. These preventive medical services should, of course, be provided in close linkage with adequate follow-up of matters requiring attention, and ideally as part of a comprehensive personal health services system. Preventive medicine consists of those physical and counseling procedures in medicine that are specifically directed toward the prevention of disease. The scope of preventive medicine thus depends first upon how one defines medicine. For example, immunization against specific diseases as a preventive measure is clearly an aspect of medicine. Other measures aimed at preventing disease are sometimes included implicitly or explicitly within the scope of "preventive medicine," for example, fluoridation of public water supplies and mass education about cigarette smoking. The latter types of disease control efforts, however, will not be included here because they fall outside the scope of medicine as defined here. For the purposes of this paper, only those preventive measures that are capable of being incorporated into personal health services will be considered. Thus, a rather strict definition of medicine is adopted.

Obviously many other activities, particularly environmental control measures and mass health education, can be effective in preventing disease. Socioeconomic advances may be the most powerful instrument of all. Socioeconomic differences in the population of the United States are a continuing influence on health, both through the level of living permitted various groups and access to medical care. None of these, however—important as they are—fall within the definition of preventive medicine in personal health services to be used here.

Secondly, the scope of preventive medicine depends upon one's view of what constitutes prevention. The narrowest interpretation would limit

2

the term to measures which prevent the actual occurrence of disease, for example, vaccination against poliomyelitis. Such measures are often called "primary prevention." A somewhat broader view includes "secondary prevention," i.e., the detection of disease in its early (asymptomatic) stages and intervention to arrest the progress of disease. This aspect of preventive medicine is well exemplified in the application of mammography for detection of breast cancer, followed by any necessary treatment. Both primary and secondary prevention imply an aggressive approach to the whole population being served. Steps are taken to reach people, to identify need for intervention, and to intervene before people present themselves for personal health services because of symptoms or other complaints.

The term "tertiary prevention" is sometimes used for efforts to maintain a maximum level of independence and activity in the chronically ill. It consists of the continuous application of measures that will restrain the progress of disease once the disease has manifested itself, for example, the continuing care of patients with decompensated heart disease. This type of health service maintenance for the chronically ill is to be differentiated from the episodic care of illness at the initiation of the patient, but it is closely allied with medical care (personal health service) in the ordinary sense. It is not included in the definition of preventive medicine for purposes of this report.

Preventive medicine, both primary and secondary, requires organization of personal health services. This may occur in the physician's office or clinic, or in some other place of care in the community such as school or place of work. The focus is on a population—either the whole population being served by a personal health service system; or some segment of it at special risk. Activity is directed not only at the patients who have come for care, but also at the rest of the population, specifically including the "nonusers" who may be in need of preventive services but do not take the initiative in seeking them. The physician and other health providers concerned with the health of the entire community must consider individuals who do not use preventive or therapeutic service as well as individuals who do.

It is in this focus on populations that preventive medicine differs most from the traditional and usual practice of medicine. Traditional medicine relies on a complaint-response system. Typically, the patient recognizes some symptom, a "complaint"; the doctor responds with diagnosis and necessary treatment. Preventive medicine, however, goes beyond these limits and adopts a health maintenance point of view. The aim is not just to respond appropriately to patients' complaints but to prevent disease and its progress by reaching out into the community. The point is that intervention in the natural history of disease is more likely to

3

be effective if it is initiated early, even before symptoms occur, than is care after full-blown pathology becomes established.

Obviously, effective preventive medicine in this sense requires a collaborative effort on the part of personal health service providers and the people being served. Responsibility for getting immunized or screened by mammography falls on the individual. That fact does not, however, relieve the health care system and its providers from a comparable responsibility for assuring that persons who seek personal health services in that system actually receive the benefits of preventive medicine. The system should involve people in taking the initiative necessary for preventive care. How people relate to the personal health service delivery system and how that system is organized determine in large part how effective preventive medicine can be. Just as individuals can be categorized with respect to their propensity to obtain preventive services, so health service systems can be categorized with respect to how fully they actually provide preventive services. Some systems of health service favor prevention more than other systems.

One side of the relationship is whether people do what is necessary for disease control, as seen from within the health care delivery system. This is sometimes called "compliance," for example, with advice to stop cigarette smoking. Clearly, such health-related behavior may reflect factors other than a physician's advice. It may be influenced also by general education, the individual's level of concern about health and life situation including exposure to peer pressures. The extent to which health-related behavior, however, is and can be influenced by contact with the personal health service delivery system is included in the concept of preventive medicine used in this paper. Seeking health behavior that will prevent disease is as much the physician's job as is seeking immunity status that will prevent disease.

Another side of the relationship is the extent to which the health care delivery system is responsive to what people want in the system, especially what they want in the way of preventive medicine. It appears now that people are beginning to recognize that more could be and should be accomplished through preventive medicine than is being accomplished. Desire for more complete application of available means for prevention of disease seems to be growing, along with demand for use of science and technology in human betterment generally. One view of this matter has been well expressed by A.W. Benn, "Technical Power and People: The Impact of Technology on the Structure of Government," *Bulletin of the Atomic Scientists* 27: 23–26, 1971.

> Now, all of a sudden, people have awakened to the fact that science and technology are just the latest expression of power and that those who control them have become the new bosses, exactly as the feudal

landlords who owned the land, or the capitalist pioneers who owned the factories, became the bosses of earlier generations. Ordinary people will not now be satisfied until they have got their hands on this power and have turned it to meet their needs.

This may sound like a very revolutionary doctrine, and so indeed it is. But once we understand what is happening, it is no more frightening than the demand for power that emerged in the past as a popular clamor for political democracy.

What we lack are the institutions capable of realizing that demand in today's world, and making it effective.

To incorporate preventive medicine systematically and completely into personal health services will require substantial modification of the present system of health care delivery.

First, it will entail reorientation of medical and related health professional education, especially a broadening of the present focus on episodic patient care to include a sense of responsibility for health maintenance. Closely related to this broader view of the purpose of personal health care is the necessity of cultivating a concern for the health of a defined population, as well as the care of individual patients. The physician should feel as guilty about a case of measles occurring in a population for whose health care he assumes responsibility as he does about missing an obvious diagnosis of appendicitis.

Further, the complete incorporation of preventive medicine into health care will entail a shift in emphasis in organized payment for personal health services. That shift will be away from what is commonly called health insurance (but is really sickness insurance), toward organized payment for health maintenance procedures. Many so-called health insurance contracts now exclude services "not medically necessary for the diagnosis or treatment of an illness or injury" and often specifically exclude certain preventive services.

Such provisions of the present organized arrangements for payment for health care must be altered so as to encourage, not discourage, preventive medical services. Also, careful consideration should be given to the organization of personal health services. Are they better provided by individual practitioners or by groups of practitioners? Should they be arranged mainly for care of episodes of illness, or mainly for health maintenance of a defined population?

This reorientation toward preventive services has, in fact, been emerging within medicine during recent decades. It has been particularly evident in the care of children and pregnant women. Pediatricians and obstetricians are directing their practices more and more toward health maintenance, and this shift is currently spreading into other branches of primary care including general internal medicine and family medicine.

5

Preventive medicine may take a variety of forms:

1. immunizing a child against communicable diseases;
2. counseling an adolescent about cigarette smoking, venereal disease, unwanted pregnancy, and use of alcohol or drugs;
3. ascertaining and treating preeclampsia in a pregnant woman;
4. detecting through amniocentesis the likelihood of a defective child and offering the mother the opportunity for abortion;
5. finding evidence of PKU in a newborn child and providing available treatment;
6. detecting and treating cervix carcinoma-in-situ in young women and breast cancer in middle-aged women; and
7. detecting and reducing elevated blood pressure in middle-aged and older men.

Preventive medicine may be focused on special population groups, such as children or young adult workers, or older people; it may be applied from the standpoint of special disease problems, such as genetic disease or cardiovascular disease; it may be approached through special groups of providers, such as pediatricians, public health nurses, or school

Table 1.   A Strategy for Improvement of Health

HEALTH PROBLEM	PERSONAL HEALTH SERVICES	ENVIRONMENTAL MEASURES	EDUCATIONAL MEASURES
Trauma from automobile accidents	Ambulance and first aid service Emergency medical service Definitive medical care and rehabilitation	Construction of streets and highways Design and construction of automobiles Road signs	Driver training Avoidance of alcohol and other drugs before driving Avoidance of driving when fatigued or upset.
Dental caries	Dental care	Fluoridation Reduce production and promotion of refined carbohydrates	Prudent diet Brush teeth
Myocardial infarction	Screen for risk factors Ambulance service Coronary care units	Alter food supply to reduce intake of foods that raise blood-cholesterol level	Exercise Prudent diet Stop cigarette smoking
Lung cancer	Detect and treat disease early	Reduce occupational exposures that cause lung cancer Reduce production and promotion of cigarettes	Stop cigarette smoking
Infant deaths	Routine pediatric care	Maintain hygiene in home Assure safe water supply	Good diet Proper mothering

nurses; it may involve special health service organizations, for example, suicide prevention organizations.

Finally, it is important to bear in mind that preventive medicine is really only one element of a larger strategy for the improvement of health. This larger approach and the place of personal health services (including both therapeutic and preventive services) in that strategy may be illustrated in Table 1.

Thus, preventive medicine, in this report, includes those aspects of personal health services that are specifically directed toward prevention of disease. It may be primary or secondary; it is focused on a population, and thus requires organization; it may take a variety of forms, but is only one element of a larger strategy to improve health.

II. Rationale

Changing Nature of Health Problems

The nature of preventive medical services, what to do to prevent disease, changes with the nature of health problems and with the scientific base for attacking these problems.

During the 19th and early 20th century the major health problem of the United States was communicable disease. It is still the major health problem in many parts of the world, affecting people mainly in the early years of life. Means of dealing with the problem include immunization; breaking the chain of infection through environmental measures, such as water sanitation; and finding and treating infected persons, for example, those with tuberculosis.

By the mid-twentieth century, however, the major health problem in the United States had come to be chronic diseases, such as heart disease and cancer, which typically and most heavily affect people after age 45. Table 2 and Fig. 1 present data illustrating the change in the nature of the health problem between 1900 and 1973, expressed as longevity, i.e., the average number of years of life remaining at various times during life. Thus, at birth a white male in the United States (death registration states) in 1900 could be expected to live on the average 48.2 years; by 1973 this had increased to 68.4 years. For all other males (mostly black), the corresponding figures were 32.5 and 61.9. Thus, there has been a more rapid rate of improvement among nonwhite males but their longevity still lags behind that of white males.

Inspection of the data reveals that a substantial portion of the gain in longevity between 1900 and 1973 was made during infancy. About half of the total gain was made during the first five years of life, and almost all the remainder during the years prior to age 45. For white males at age 45, the gain in longevity—considering all advances in medical science and levels of living—was less than four years; and for other males the gain was less than five years. Females gained about nine years in longevity after age 45.

The relatively small gain after age 45, especially for males, reflects two facts. One is that heart disease and cancer cause death mainly after that age, and progress against those diseases has been slow. The principal advances in preventive medicine (and health) have been against the communicable diseases in early life. The other fact is that certain forms of cancer and heart disease have actually increased substantially since 1900, especially lung cancer and coronary heart disease.

Thus the health problem in the United States has changed remarkably since the beginning of the century. Now heart disease and cancer are

Table 2

AGE, RACE, AND SEX	AVERAGE NUMBER OF YEARS OF LIFE REMAINING	
	1973	1900–1902
White Males		
0	68.4	48.23
1	68.6	54.61
5	64.9	54.43
45	27.8	24.21
All Other Males		
0	61.9	32.54
1	62.8	42.46
5	59.1	45.06
45	24.9	20.09
White Females		
0	76.1	51.08
1	76.1	56.39
5	72.3	56.03
45	33.9	25.51
All Other Females		
0	70.1	35.04
1	70.8	43.54
5	67.1	46.04
45	30.3	21.36

Source: National Center for Health Statistics, *Life Tables, Vital Statistics of the United States 1973,* Volume II, Section 5. U.S. Government Printing Office, 1975.

the main causes of death (and considerable disability), and these deaths begin to weigh most heavily after age 45; formerly communicable diseases in early life were the outstanding problem.

This should not be taken to imply that communicable diseases no longer constitute a problem in the United States. They are, in fact, still a considerable burden on the population. Nor should one assume that progress against disease in infancy has been so great that little more will occur. In fact, the rate of infant mortality in the United States remained stationary from 1955–1965 and then began to decline in the late 1960s. It is still higher in the United States than in several other countries and could in all likelihood be substantially reduced.

By mid-twentieth century, however, the major health problem in the United States had clearly come to be the chronic diseases of middle and later life.

Lung cancer and coronary heart disease require a much different approach from that developed against typhoid fever and poliomyelitis. In the present state of knowledge, dealing preventively with chronic disease consists to a considerable extent of identifying risk factors for particular conditions, for example, cigarette smoking and high blood pressure, and minimizing such risk factors in the population. Ideally, the latter should be avoided entirely. That is possible for many individuals who have not

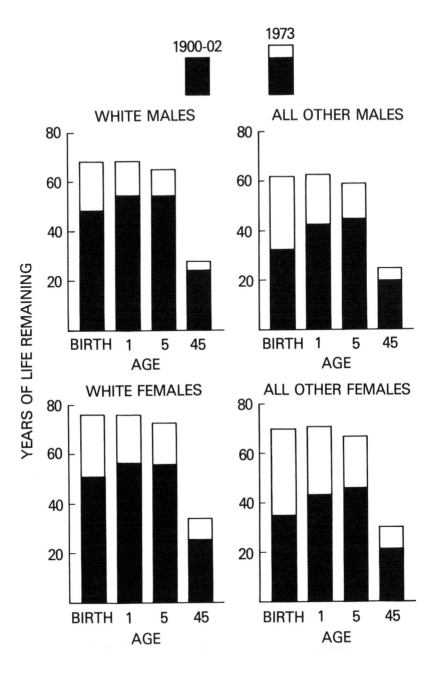

Figure 1. Average Number of Years of Life Remaining in 1973 vs. 1900–1902 for Different Age, Race, and Sex Groups.

acquired the risk factor. For other individuals, in whom the risk is already present, action must be taken to reduce it.

Measures for the control of the known risk factors for chronic disease may be specified by the physician but they must generally be adopted and carried out by the individuals concerned. Incorporating this approach into personal health services is one means of preventing the major conditions now adversely affecting health.

Empirical Basis for Preventive Medicine

An important means of preventing the health problems of our day, then, is to influence the daily habits of people. These health problems are now known to be caused largely by various aspects of a new style of life, including cigarette smoking and excessive consumption of alcohol and food, that prevails among many people in the United States. The means of dealing with the current major health problems, thus, will evidently be much more dependent on personal, life-long behavior than has been true of health problems in the past. It will be necessary to involve individuals themselves in controlling these diseases, at least in the face of our present understanding of the origin of the major chronic diseases.

Not only do personal habits play a large role in the causation of the major health problem of our day, and thus provide a basis for attacking the major chronic diseases, but scientific and technological achievements have provided another approach towards the prevention of disease. The technical means have been developed for surveillance of several aspects of human functioning that are related to the chronic diseases. Systematic observation of certain conditions in man permits the identification of deviations that often evolve into the abnormalities that we call diseases.

For example, higher diastolic and/or systolic blood pressure than "normal" may be a precursor of hypertension and the diseases associated with that condition. Evidence is now accumulating to indicate that finding and treating people with blood pressure at levels higher than "normal" can be beneficial. The condition may otherwise progress to permanent damage, even though the blood pressure would not in previous years have been regarded as high enough (if not associated with enlargement of the heart or other abnormalities) to justify treatment. Modern treatment may avoid continued, high blood pressure levels if the condition is found early enough. If not, high blood pressure may lead to disability and premature death in a significant proportion of the hypertensive population.

Listed below are several categories of conditions that can be systematically observed in order to detect abnormalities when they can be most effectively handled.

Immunologic

Susceptibility to measles, poliomyelitis, diphtheria, pertussis, tetanus, and other infectious diseases can be ascertained by history and sometimes by other means. Artificial induction of immunity to such diseases is then indicated, with emphasis on certain time periods of life. Immunologic surveillance is now also applicable to other situations important to health, such as in Rh incompatibility between mother and fetus and in certain allergic conditions for which treatment can be effective.

Bacterial

Invasion of the body by bacteria and other organisms continues to be an important cause of disease, for example, tuberculosis, syphilis, gonorrhea, and urinary tract infections. Techniques are available for the detection of such infections. Use of these techniques is important not only for protecting the health of the individuals infected, but often for the protection of other individuals as well. Thus, surveys indicate that asymptomatic infection with gonorrhea exists to the extent of 1–5 percent in various groups of young women in whom such infection would not be suspected because of symptoms. It is becoming evident that these asymptomatic infections of young women constitute not only a hazard to such women, but also an important reservoir for the continued epidemic of gonorrhea in the United States as well as elsewhere in the world.

Anatomical

Perhaps the most widespread health-related abnormality of anatomy in the United States is excessive weight in relation to height. For years it has been well recognized that excessive weight, at least in many population groups, carries a risk of morbidity and mortality higher than that among individuals of the same group who have a normal weight-height relationship. Lumps of a certain character in the breast also are being recognized as early cancer, through physical examination by physicians, through self-examination and by mammography. Microscopic examination of scrapings from the cervix can reveal early abnormalities called cervical dysplasia or carcinoma-in-situ; if not corrected, they may eventuate in cancer of the uterus and fatality. Dental caries and disorders are another widespread anatomical abnormality which can be frequently prevented through prophylaxis or discovered early and corrected with avoidance of future morbidity; if neglected, these lesions may result in loss of teeth or other harm. Other conditions for which routine surveillance is useful include congenital dislocation of the hip and congenital heart disease.

12

Physiological

Elevated blood pressure has already been mentioned. Excessive intraocular tension can likewise be detected, often an early evidence of the onset of the disease glaucoma, but it is not clear that loss of vision can be avoided any more completely by treatment during the stage when the condition can be discovered by screening than later when symptoms first occur. Loss of visual or auditory acuity may indicate the need for intervention before the individual has any sense that disease is occurring. Abnormalities detected by electrocardiography are now routinely sought by many internists, particularly in susceptible individuals, with a view toward instituting measures for avoiding the effects of coronary heart disease.

Chemical

High blood cholesterol is generally recognized as an important risk factor in coronary heart disease. The precise value of lowering blood cholesterol as a preventive measure for that disease is being actively investigated. Likewise it is clear that diabetes can be detected in its early stages, before the onset of symptoms, through measurement of blood glucose; treatment of the condition by dietary means (and avoiding the use of drugs) can be helpful. Measurement of hemoglobin or hematocrit is performed in many circumstances for the purpose of initiating any indicated treatment to maintain normal hemoglobin level and thus facilitate the maintenance of health. Increased urinary protein and sugar are other examples of abnormalities that can be detected readily in a chemical approach to health maintenance.

Behaviorial

Cigarette smoking in the United States and in many other countries is clearly a habit with profoundly adverse effect on health. Excessive use of alcohol and other drugs is common throughout the world where people are affluent enough to gain access to as much of these substances as they desire. Excessive use arising from complex motivation can lead to severe degrees of ill health and early mortality. Besides the adverse effect of using cigarettes, alcohol, and other substances with harmful effects, states of anxiety, depression, and other emotional disorders that are evident in behavior likewise may portend harm to health.

Inspection of the above list, and it could be considerably more detailed, suggests that routine surveillance of various parameters of human function may be useful in detecting abnormalities before they are ordinarily recognized and when intervention may be most effective.

Additional items or refinements of existing ones, are being proposed for incorporation into the outline given above. For example, investigators are now actively exploring other chemical measures as signals of incipient disease and the precise levels of blood pressure that merit active treatment.

These and dozens of other procedures for detecting abnormal conditions must still be further evaluated to determine the extent of their usefulness, particularly the value of intervention after finding the abnormality. Still, enough is known about the periodic monitoring of such factors and about the value of correcting many abnormalities, that the technical foundation for approaching preventive medicine through routine surveillance may be regarded as established. For example, the American Heart Association has prepared a handbook that estimates the probability of developing atherothrombotic brain infarction in eight years based on several risk factors (age, sex, elevated blood pressure, ECG abnormalities, glucose intolerance, high levels of serum cholesterol, the cigarette smoking habit). The handbook can thus be used as a guide in the selection of stroke candidates for preventive management. It is stated that preventive measures available for modification of the major stroke precursors include antihypertension agents, antiarrhythmic drugs, anticoagulants, and carotid artery surgery; and that the use of these corrective measures appears reasonable in high risk stroke candidates even though the proof of efficacy has not been established for all.

Knowledge has advanced to the point that it is possible to list many specific procedures that should be carried out at particular times of life to protect health. On the other hand, many of the procedures proposed are as yet in various stages of being tested, or further developed, with a view toward routine application in personal health services if definite benefits can be proved.

It is important to emphasize that this approach to preventive medicine at the present time serves only to alert the physician to the possibility of damage to health that may be occurring. Some abnormality can be discovered in just about everyone, and it is obviously unwise to turn everyone into a "patient." Further, it is important to avoid the possible adverse effects of the screening procedures themselves, for example, the use of radiation in mammography. Finally, it must be recognized that there are large areas potentially important for preventive medicine where our knowledge is grossly inadequate. The present state of medical science can do little to relieve the burden of much chronic illness, for example, in the mental health field and in rheumatic disease.

Technical achievements, however, continue to bring promise of providing insight into the natural history of disease, especially pinpointing where disease may be most vulnerable to preventive measures.

Thus the electron microscope has provided the capability of detecting changes at the cellular level, and biochemistry has yielded techniques for measuring enzyme levels, that may be useful in preventive medicine. Emphasis should be placed on using such developments in basic science to explore cellular and enzymatic changes that may be precursors of disease, detectable at a time when intervention could be most effective. In this connection, it should be noted that the rate of change in the individual is important as well as the existence of abnormal conditions.

Theoretical Basis for Preventive Medicine

The future advance of preventive medicine may lie substantially in linking basic science more directly with epidemiology. The clinician will serve as the intervening interpretor of the disease significance of what is disclosed through basic science research, and help to judge the effectiveness of intervention in situations that cannot yet be regarded as disease. The basic scientist in immunology, physiology, anatomy, and other fields may, however, now profitably join the epidemiologist in elucidating the mechanisms and early stages of disease that can lead to preventive measures.

Important as is this approach to preventive medicine, it must be emphasized that the science of epidemiology has made significant contributions to understanding of disease even in the absence of insight into disease mechanisms. This has been true from the time that James Lind discovered the cause of scurvy to be the absence of citrus fruit, or other sources of vitamin C as later noted; through the time when John Snow discovered the cause of cholera to be polluted water, prior to the establishment of the idea of bacterial cause of disease; down to the discovery that cigarette smoking causes lung cancer, without understanding exactly how this happens.

Personal health care has been and still is essentially a complaint-response system. The patient brings his complaint to a physician who responds by making a diagnosis and prescribing or carrying out therapy. The purpose is to resolve the patient's complaint. The complaint-response system generally works quite well for the patient who has a severe pain in the abdomen or other serious symptoms. It is, however, increasingly recognized as insufficient for complete health care whose intent is to avoid premature death and unnecessary disability. Complaints need an appropriate response, but the presentation and handling of them can be more effective as part of a larger health-maintenance system of care.

An orientation towards restoring, maintaining, and protecting optimal function is a fundamental aspect of the preventive approach in personal health care. Thus, responding to an episode of cardiac decompensation by brief hospitalization of the patient and discharge with a prescription is not sufficient. In order really to protect optimal functioning, it will often be necessary to provide continuing care. For example, a public health nurse or other health worker may visit the patient's home after discharge with congestive heart failure to assist the patient in following the regime prescribed, rather than simply waiting for another episode of decompensation to occur and bring the patient back to the hospital. Continuing and comprehensive care of such patients is necessary for best results. While seemingly close to what most physicians do in their care of patients with chronic illness, the difference in emphasis and point of view is extremely important.

On the one hand the physician waits for the presentation of complaints and responds with an episode of care, either in the office, clinic or hospital. From then on, the responsibility is totally that of the patient. The physician and the health care delivery system simply await further developments.

The preventive orientation, on the other hand, is to continue the care wherever and however it might be needed so as to preserve, maintain, and protect optimal function.

The incorporation of preventive medicine into personal health services may be regarded as deliberately and regularly adding primary and secondary preventive procedures to a system of comprehensive, continuing health care of all persons in the population. It will obviously entail a change in orientation and a change in the organization of personal health care services.

Dynamic Nature of Preventive Medicine

Effectively revising the personal health service delivery system to incorporate preventive medical services more systematically requires that attention be given to the dynamic nature of preventive medicine itself. Provision should be made for adding new procedures as they are developed, evaluated and judged ready for general application. For example, care during pregnancy is designed not only to protect the health of the woman but also to assure the birth of a healthy infant. A new technique, amniocentesis, has been developed as a means of detecting Down's syndrome (a common cause of mental retardation) and other conditions likely to result in a deformed fetus. Within a relatively short time routine application of amniocentesis in pregnancy, especially among older women, may be recognized as desirable. Some would say the time has already arrived. Whenever a preventive technique has been found useful, it should be made available generally in the health services delivery system.

16

The incorporation of amniocentesis into the health services delivery system, however, should be arranged with a view not only to its present application in Down's syndrome and a few other conditions, but also with a view toward its possible expansion for the detection of additional conditions that may result in a deformed or dead fetus. The current rapid advances in medical science, including those in genetics, make it likely that preventive medicine using such techniques as amniocentesis will move ahead rapidly in coming years.

The recent history of preventive medicine indicates that it often takes 5–25 years for a technique once developed to be widely applied in health care. The personal health services delivery system must become more responsive to innovations in preventive medicine. Lag between development and general use should be reduced by more prompt and systematic evaluation of new procedures—followed, if they are found meritorious, by rapid incorporation into routine care. Only then will the potential of preventive medicine be fully realized.

Once a framework for providing preventive medical services is established, it should be carefully watched to assure that new advances are promptly incorporated, unnecessary or harmful procedures weeded out, and adjustment made in the system of preventive medicine itself whenever it is found wanting.

Probably the most difficult aspect of properly incorporating preventive medicine into personal health services is the determination of precisely what conditions are to be prevented, by what procedures, by what means and at what cost. Objectives should be explicitedly stated. Expectations must be made clear, not only to those involved in health services administration and in health care professional work, but also to the general public. This should be done, condition by condition, and procedure by procedure, to the maximum extent possible. It is essential to minimize the hazard of false hope, as well as to minimize unnecessary delay in the application of procedures that have been found to yield benefits. The following two sections will deal with these issues in greater depth.

III. Application

History

Probably the outstanding achievement of preventive medicine has been the control of several major communicable diseases through immunization as a means of primary prevention. Smallpox, which killed millions throughout the world and remained a threat to the United States until recent years, is now rapidly being eliminated from the face of the earth. Only remote villages in a few countries remain infected and 1975 may see the last cases of the disease; if so, it will be the first major disease to be completely conquered. Diphtheria, a scourge of infants and young children only a few decades ago, has been reduced to isolated cases and small outbreaks in the United States. Poliomyelitis, which still was striking this nation with great force only a quarter-century ago, has been virtually eliminated. Measles, pertussis, tetanus, and other diseases for which immunizing agents have been developed likewise have been vastly reduced in frequency.

While taking pride in these advances in disease control through primary prevention, two points deserve emphasis. One is that, with the possible exception of poliomyelitis for which the preventive medicine procedure was applied effectively within a very few years, the other important communicable diseases were tolerated for many years after control measures became available. Some are still tolerated. Our failure to eliminate measles in the United States, even 10 years after the technical means were available, highlights the problems of personal health service in this country that hinder preventive medicine. The second point is the continuing need for vigilance in both observing the occurrence of disease that can be controlled by immunization, with prompt response to outbreaks; and maintaining sufficiently high levels of immunity in communities irrespective of disease occurrence. Experience with measles indicates the danger of relaxing effort when the job is incomplete.

The idea and practice of secondary prevention came into being during the campaigns against tuberculosis and syphilis during the 1930s and 1940s. Early case finding through mass use of chest x-rays and blood tests, with follow-up of cases for treatment of individuals and accordance of spread, emphasized the value of dealing with disease before the classical symptoms appeared—in fact, during the asymptomatic stage of disease. In the late 1940s this same approach was extended to cancer of the cervix using the Papanicolaou smear, and to diabetes with a simple test for blood sugar level. Since those days the idea of secondary prevention has spread slowly but steadily.

One of the first, and still one of the most important, elements of prevention to be introduced was the public health nurse visit. Instead of waiting for mothers to bring their sick children into public clinics, health departments and visiting nurse associations launched a system of having nurses visit homes. There they reinforced the advice given in the clinics, gave practical lessons to the mother in carrying out indicated procedures, observed and sought to correct home conditions contributing to ill health and arranged necessary return visits to the clinic. This same approach was also applied to other conditions such as tuberculosis and more recently other chronic diseases.

These early efforts in preventive medicine focused on specific population groups with particular problems that could be tackled with the means of primary or secondary prevention then available. Pregnant women, infants and preschool children were among the first beneficiaries. Recently preventive medicine of essentially the same kind has been spreading further into medicine as a whole. Family physicians, general internists, and other primary care physicians are beginning to adopt this orientation for their practices involving the population as a whole. While still spotty in application and by no means having replaced episodic care as the general pattern, preventive medicine is making some headway beyond its traditional role.

Factors Influencing Expansion of Preventive Medicine

Several major forces influence the expansion of preventive medicine in personal health services.

Probably the fundamental force is scientific and technical advance. Actually having the means to prevent disease obviously is the sine qua non and gives thrust to application for human benefit. Hence preventive medicine must constantly encourage research and development toward ever more effective means of disease prevention as an essential element in realizing the full potential of the field. To this end epidemiology must be encouraged, especially in association with physiology, immunology, and the other basic science fields in which fundamental progress may yield new clues to disease control.

Another key factor in the application of preventive medicine lies in the attitudes, knowledge, and practices of health care providers. Health professional, and especially medical, education still emphasizes and reinforces an orientation toward the diagnosis and treatment of disease brought by patients to medical centers and their clinics where medical and related education is concentrated. This emphasis undoubtedly prepares physicians and others to deal effectively with manifestations of disease, but the almost exclusive preoccupation with that aspect of medicine leaves little time or encouragement for the preventive approach. The sense of responsibility for health maintenance is not sufficiently cultivated. Thus a major problem in the application of preventive medicine is to reorient more rapidly than seems to be occurring the attitudes and practices of physicians and other health care providers through health professional education.

At present the general public appears as ready as, perhaps more ready than, the health professions to embrace preventive medicine as an important part of personal medical services. Executives of major companies are commonly provided, and take advantage of, periodic medical examinations directed toward health maintenance; these are often a part of their company "fringe benefits" and looked upon favorably both by management and by the individuals involved. The check-ups received by the President of the United States are well publicized. About 1950 the International Longshoremen and Warehousemen's Union in the San Francisco Bay Area insisted upon organized medical check-ups by the Kaiser Health Plan, enforcing a contract that provided such services. Subsequently the union representing cannery workers in California negotiated with employers an ear-marked fund for examinations directed toward preventive medicine, to be provided through a mobile unit visiting the cannery plants in several counties of the state. Recently, construction workers in Hawaii have negotiated periodic health examinations into their contract with employers, and further to have these examinations organized through the Blue Shield Plan of Hawaii by groups of physicians willing to take on the task.

This enthusiasm of consumer groups for preventive medicine may, of course, sometimes be misdirected because of inadequate technical knowledge. Greatly needed at present are channels of communication between those competent in the technical aspects of preventive medicine and the increasingly sophisticated union and other groups that want modern preventive medicine on an organized basis for their members. Observation of what executives and political leaders are getting in the way of preventive medicine apparently is not without some effect on their thinking.

How personal health services are organized can have a major impact on the extent to which preventive features are incorporated. Studies have demonstrated that prepaid group practice plans actually do provide such services as the Papanicolaou smear and examinations directed toward health maintenance to a greater extent than these services are provided for comparable groups who subscribe to other health care plans.

A preventive services index applied to comparable groups of subscribers to group practice plans, provider plans and commercial plans in Southern California showed that persons in the group practice plans had received a higher level of services defined as preventive than had persons in the other types of plans. It thus seems evident that group-practice prepayment plans do offer an advantage over the traditional method of arranging personal health services, insofar as preventive medicine is concerned. The organization of care appears to be a key element.

The nature of financing health care also exerts a substantial influence on how preventive services are actually used. As noted earlier, many sickness ("health") insurance plans specifically exclude such services from the plan benefits. The use of so-called coinsurance, in the form of deductibles and partial payment by patients at the time of service, has been advocated as a means of deterring "excessive" use of medical care; that principle has been incorporated into many current insurance plans and proposed in certain national health insurance plans. Opponents have insisted that such copayment deters especially poor people from obtaining needed early care and preventive services. Some interesting evidence on this point has recently come from a study of patients receiving Medi-Caid services in California; it showed that when copayment is required it exerts a major adverse effect on obtaining preventive services. The latter are actually used much less frequently when copayment is required.

Current Extent of Application

As stated earlier, preventive medicine may be viewed as a composite of many types of preventive activity. Prevention to avoid the occurrence of disease may be interpreted as including such things as legislation, education of the public, nutrition, occupational safety, fire prevention, highway safety, environmental control of carcinogens, regular exercise, immunization, and avoiding cigarette smoking or excessive alcohol. Prevention thus embraces by a wide diversity of effort, both within and outside the realm of personal health service. The purpose of this section, however, is to identify illustrative, major preventive activities that may be provided within the personal health service system.

Personal education and counseling by the physician or his associates is certainly a major component of primary prevention. The aim is the prevention of disease, particularly chronic disease, through influencing an individual's lifestyle. Examples include:

1. Modification of diet to reduce intake of sweets, saturated fat and cholesterol;
2. Exercise to combat physical inactivity;
3. Cessation of cigarette smoking;
4. Reduction in the consumption of alcohol;
5. Reduction of obesity;

6. Genetic counseling and family planning;
7. Nutritional practices;
8. Accident prevention.

Another major element of primary prevention is prophylaxis. Immunoprophylaxis for infectious diseases, as noted above, has been the most successful application of preventive medicine with proven substantial results.

Currently immunizations are provided for the prevention of diphtheria, tetanus, pertussis, poliomyelitis, measles, mumps, and rubella. Until recently smallpox immunizations were also routinely given. Now smallpox immunization is provided selectively, along with influenza immunizations. Other applications of prophylaxis include use of silver nitrate for prevention of gonorrheal ophthalmia in newborns, and anti-Rh-immune globulin in appropriate situations to prevent infant mortality.

Secondary prevention of various conditions through screening followed by early treatment is of particular importance in reducing morbidity and mortality due to chronic diseases and disorders. Numerous screening procedures are presently being utilized. Because of cost considerations and the infrequency with which individual conditions occur in the general population, screening is generally directed toward specific high risk groups:

1. Screening of Rh-negative mothers for the presence of antibodies;
2. Screening for bacteriuria in pregnancy;
3. Ultrasonic scanning for determination of fetal growth;
4. Detection of fetal chromosome abnormalities in older pregnant women through transabdominal amniocentesis;
5. Screening for phenylketonuria and other inherited metabolic diseases in new-born infants;
6. Screening of infants for development and growth malformations such as mental retardation or specific diseases such as congenital hip instability and cardiovascular disease;
7. Screening of children for abnormalities of hearing and vision, communicative disorders and learning disabilities;
8. Screening for cardiovascular disease by detection of high blood pressure and elevated blood lipids such as cholesterol and triglycerides;
9. Screening for pulmonary tuberculosis;
10. Detection of cervical dysplasia and breast lesions;
11. Screening for gonorrhea by cervical culture and serological testing for syphilis;
12. Identification of cases of diabetes responsive to therapy;
13. Screening four-to-five year old females for bacteruria followed by examination for anatomic defects in persistent cases.

22

These screening procedures are frequently carried out as single tests in specific high risk groups or individuals. Another approach to secondary prevention involves the simultaneous use of a battery of multiple tests. There are a variety of multiphasic or multiple test programs in existence, each with a different number and combination of tests. The specific tests included in each program depend on a host of program design and population considerations. Multiphasic screening frequently includes several of the following: electrocardiogram, blood pressure, chest x-ray, spirometry, anthropometry, skin-fold thickness, hearing and vision tests, tonometry, retinal photography, serological test for syphilis, cervical cytology, breast palpation, mammography, thermography, proctosigmoidoscopy, psychometrics, achilleometry, dental exam, and dental x-ray.

An overview of the present use of preventive medicine in personal health services can also be obtained by identifying the conditions or diseases which are to prevented. Since the current emphasis in medicine is on diseases this may be an appropriate summary format.

Infectious disease control includes therapeutic control of respiratory virus and bacterial infections such as streptococcal disease and pneumococcal pneumonia; population surveillance of gonorrhea by cervical culture and prompt treatment of contacts of identified carriers, as well as prophylaxis of gonorrheal ophthalmia in newborns; surveillance of human carriers and treatment with gamma globulin for infectious hepatitis; and immunizations for diphtheria, tetanus, pertussis, poliomyelitis, measles, mumps, and rubella.

Reduction of cardiovascular disease is carried out through modification of major risk factors including blood cholesterol, blood pressure, and cigarette smoking. Detection of cardiovascular system abnormalities followed by treatment is also an important part of preventive medicine.

Renal disease is controlled through detection and treatment of hypertension; screening groups at high risk for pyelonephritis; screening tests for blood-urea nitrogen and creatinine; urinalysis and early treatment of diabetes.

Prevention of complications of diabetes and its associated vascular disease is uncertain. Therapy aimed at the control of blood glucose levels has been disappointing.

Detection of pulmonary tuberculosis is the target of the tuberculin skin test and the chest x-ray. Spirometry has also been used to detect abnormal respiratory function. The chest x-ray and sputum cytology are used to detect lung cancer.

Cancer is detected through the application of various screening procedures aimed at abnormal cervical cells, breast lesions, occult blood in stool, abnormal chest x-ray, and lesions of the colon.

Prevention of fetal and neonatal mortality is carried out by: family planning and counseling of the pregnant mother; monitoring of the mother and intrauterine monitoring of the fetus; and intensive care neonatal units.

Dental caries and periodontal disease may be partially controlled through prophylactic dental care, including counseling on diet and oral hygiene.

Principles of Application

With current progress in preventive medicine, certain principles are beginning to emerge:

1. Periodic evaluation of the disease problems in a community and the means for dealing with these problems in an optimally effective manner is necessary.

2. Health care providers must be kept informed about what is happening in the community that affects preventive medicine.

3. It is essential to make explicit to the general public the benefits and the limitations of preventive medicine.

4. Several parties, including individual members of the public as well as the system of personal health services, carry responsibility for achieving the benefits of preventive medicine.

5. More attention should be given to the prevention of chronic illness in middle and later years through action during the early years of life. For example, the prevention of certain forms of chronic lung disease involves preventive measures starting in infancy. To prevent those forms of cardiovascular disease linked with hypertension it now appears desirable to start with teenage groups. Alcoholism and cervix cancer as well as lung cancer likewise appear increasingly to have their roots in the teenage period of life. Waiting until 40, or even until 30, years of age may be too late.

6. A single procedure may be effective against several conditions. For example, control of cigarette smoking can be effective not only against lung cancer but also against coronary heart disease. In fact, more deaths from coronary heart disease than lung cancer may be avoided through control of cigarette smoking.

7. A considerable amount of preventable disease still arises from occupational exposure. Even though social reform has improved conditions in the work place during recent decades, technological advances that are being incorporated into industry generate new hazards to health. Constant vigilance is necessary to avoid man-made disease in the work place.

8. Preventive medicine may be carried out as an element of personal health service in a variety of places: office, clinic, industry, school, health

center, and other places. Careful attention must be given to the most effective ways and places in which preventive medicine can be delivered. One pattern may be most effective for one condition or one group of people, but other patterns may be more effective for others.

9. Designating responsibility for a certain population (for example, those living in a geographically defined area or enrolled in a certain health care plan) can be a highly potent force in achieving application of preventive medicine procedures. This factor may be of major significance in influencing health care professionals and organizations for the delivery of health care toward preventive medicine. Organization is certainly essential in encouraging the incorporation of preventive medical procedures into personal health services and insuring that everyone is in the system with access to preventive medicine.

10. Unified financing is necessary for the development of effective preventive medical services. The fragmentation of financing into separate pieces—for various groups of the population, for various places of care, and for various conditions—loosens responsibility for the comprehensive health care of individuals including health maintenance measures. At the time unified financing is achieved, however, it is essential that high priority be given to preventive medicine; otherwise the tendency for preventive medicine to be played down in relation to the demands for care of acute illness may simply be more firmly established.

11. Further research is necessary to develop more fully the theory and application of preventive medicine in personal health services. Such research should be conducted in the context of a strategy for health improvement involving all three major elements of such improvement: personal health services; environmental control measures; and means of influencing health-related behavior.

12. Research to advance preventive medicine should be directed in considerable part toward elucidating natural history of diseases. Such knowledge indicates the most vulnerable points in disease development, where intervention may be effective. Examining the present state of medical science in relation to the natural history of diseases will indicate the potential as well as directions, through research endeavor, of establishing more effective intervention. This approach to research in preventive medicine should not, of course, be taken to imply any curtailment of biologic research and social research in general, from which leads might be found for improving health.

13. While research is the fundamental way to enhance our capability in preventive medicine, the application of knowledge derived from research must always be based on prudence. Preventive medical procedures should be tested not only on individuals but also for community effectiveness; possible ill, as well as good effect; and relationship to other

means for the control of diseases. Prudence involves the timeliness and extent of application which is justifiable on rational grounds, at various times in the development of knowledge. For some procedures directed towards certain conditions, one would want to have complete scientific proof of effectiveness and relative harmlessness; for other procedures and conditions something less than absolute scientific knowledge may be sufficient to justify action.

IV. Issues

Orientation Toward Conditions

In the further development of preventive medicine as an aspect of personal health services, several issues must be faced.

First is the matter of defining what is to be prevented, and what is to be the basis for proceeding. While the general aim, of course, is to prevent diseases that cause substantial morbidity and mortality in the population, it now appears desirable to focus on *conditions that lead to diseases.* Conditions that are often precursors to full-blown diseases become the target. Action should be directed toward susceptibility to disease that can be overcome by immunization, toward high blood pressure and carcinoma-in-situ before these conditions have developed into symptomatic disease. It is these types of conditions that often precede morbidity and mortality that have become the immediate concern of preventive medicine.

These conditions are to be approached preventively through a wide range of activities in personal health services. The emphasis is not so much on the particular procedures that are known to be useful, and possibly could even be expanded in usefulness, but on the conditions against which the whole of preventive medicine is to be mobilized. This emphasis is a truly comprehensive one, not limited to sentinel diseases, nor to particular procedures—however effective and fashionable they may be. Preventive medicine calls for a broad reorientation of health care, not merely campaigns against particular diseases and the application of particular procedures. Although some things are best done in campaigns, most preventive measures should be incorporated into long-term programs.

Evaluation Criteria

A second issue concerns the appropriate criteria to adopt for determining whether specific preventive procedures should be incorporated into health care services. General criteria useful in the evaluation of both primary and secondary preventive procedures include: effectiveness of the procedure; frequency and seriousness of the condition; effectiveness of other means of dealing with the condition, including routine diagnosis and treatment; feasibility of adding the procedure to present arrangements for health care; and cost. Appendix I outlines five sets of criteria that have been advanced particularly for screening and detection (secondary prevention). Drawing heavily on these criteria, a composite list has been prepared that is generally applicable in the consideration of preventive procedures. These criteria are divided into three groups: nature of condition, effectiveness of preventive procedure, and feasibility of application.

Nature of Condition

1. The condition which is the target of the preventive procedure must be clearly identified.

2. The prevalence and significance of the condition should warrant classification as an important health problem for the community.

3. The natural history of disease(s) associated with the condition should be understood sufficiently to justify intervention.

4. For secondary prevention the condition should be recognizable at an early stage.

Effectiveness of Procedure

1. The application of a preventive procedure should be known to alter favorably the natural history of the disease, with greater effect than traditional treatment methods. Modification of risk factors is helpful to know but is not final evidence of effectiveness against ultimate disease.

2. The financial gains and losses associated with the application of a preventive procedure, including subsequent intervention, if any, should be known. While certain aspects of cost can be fairly easily measured, for example, the cost of medical care and the loss of productivity, the value of life itself and the quality of life is hardly calculable in ordinary terms such as dollars.

3. Social benefits and costs ascribable to the community at large (beyond groups to be treated) should be considered.

4. Efficacy of each individual component of a preventive program should be demonstrated, and the appropriateness of combining preventive procedures must be determined; differences in distribution of target conditions in the population may render combination inappropriate.

5. Cost effectiveness of preventive procedure should exceed cost effectiveness of other available methods of preventing or treating disease. Such cost-effectiveness determinations should give consideration to all aspects of the problem, including health as well as dollars. Health gains and long-term beneficial effect, measured in improvement in end results of health such as function and survival, must outweigh detrimental effects of intervention, including labeling people as "diseased" or "high risk."

Feasibility of Application

1. There must be a clear identification of the population to receive a particular preventive procedure.

2. A preventive procedure must be applicable and acceptable to the appropriate population and easy to administer, preferably by paramedical personnel.

3. When necessary as a follow-up to the application of a preventive procedure, a suitable form of diagnostic and therapeutic intervention must exist which is applicable and acceptable to the population involved; compliance should be at a level which is effective in altering the natural history of the disease in the community.

4. Sufficient resources must be available for application of the preventive procedure, and for any diagnostic or therapeutic intervention that may be required during follow-up.

In deciding upon incorporation of preventive medical procedures into personal health services, prudence becomes a major factor. The evidence available for decision is usually imperfect; scientific skepticism is properly applicable not only toward many things that have been included in medicine for years but also toward what is new in preventive medicine.

One reason for continuing uncertainty in the minds of some experts about the value of certain procedures and the necessity of relying on judgement rather than overwhelming scientific evidence, is that we do not have the means, tradition, or system for rationally examining in desirable detail what is done or proposed in medicine. Action based on prudence prevails widely in medicine as a whole as well as in preventive medicine. Steps toward improving this situation are under way in the form of clinical trials in general medicine and mass trials in preventive medicine. For example, the current, nationwide trial of mammography, and the MRFIT program may pioneer a new tradition in this country which would vastly enhance the usefulness of preventive medicine. Meanwhile, because such trials may require years to complete and even then may not be definitive, and because for other procedures in preventive medicine such trials are not feasible, it will be necessary to make decisions on the basis of prudent evaluation of what evidence exists. Here a serious difficulty arises; agreement on the adherence to what seems prudent is not as easy as agreement on what is demonstrated with overwhelming scientific force. There is and should be a place for skepticism. Conservatism about application of procedures on a mass scale is at least as justified as when the application is to an individual patient.

On the other hand, the issue of social equity arises here. Too often the advantages of new developments in preventive medicine are first acquired by those with means and sophistication to obtain them rather

29

than those in greatest need. The recent history of preventive medicine abounds with examples of favoritism to the well-to-do extending for decades, as in the case of the Papanicolaou smear, measles immunization, and the contraceptive pill. Such social bias can hardly be justified on the basis of either science or prudence.

Social rationality and prudence must be given greater weight than heretofore in applying preventive medicine.

Assessment of Selected Preventive Medicine Procedures

Immunizations

Immunization through the administration of vaccines is now a well established part of preventive medicine. Currently vaccines can be used against diphtheria, pertussis, tetanus, smallpox, poliomyelitis, mumps, rubella, and measles. However, in considering the efficacy of vaccines along with the costs and benefits associated with their administration, it is evident that not all can be recommended as a universal, routine part of primary prevention.

Smallpox vaccination is no longer recommended as a routine. By 1968 the health cost of smallpox vaccination had become greater than its benefits in the United States. The health cost included 8,024 complications, of which 152 were major complications, with nine deaths. The benefits associated with smallpox vaccination are more difficult to determine; the last cases of smallpox in the United States were reported in 1949. Because of a greatly reduced risk of smallpox importation from another country and a reduced risk of spread in the U.S., the possible risk of the disease is clearly outweighed by the complications due to vaccination. As a result of weighing these factors, the U.S. Public Health Service and the American Academy of Pediatrics recommended in 1971 that routine vaccination against smallpox should be terminated. The control of smallpox thus represents a classic model to be followed in preventive medicine. A preventive procedure is introduced and then withdrawn when the costs of the procedure outweigh the potential remaining cost of the disease.

Immunization against pertussis also occasions some health losses in the form of vaccination reactions and rarely a more serious complication. Vaccination is still effective, however, in reducing the incidence, severity and duration of the disease. Thus the benefits of immunization are substantial in comparison with adverse effects.

Immunization against measles has been highly beneficial. Incidence has been reduced to a mere fraction of the prevaccination level and it is estimated that net benefits during the first decade of artificial immunization include an estimated 2,400 lives saved. There is little question that benefits outweigh costs. However, rather than a progressive decline in the number of measles cases leading to an eventual eradication, a resurgence of measles cases was reported in 1969 which continued into 1970 and 1971. As a result the efficacy of measles vaccine was questioned. Subsequently, it has been determined that the principal reason for this increase in measles was the failure to maintain an adequate level of immunization in the susceptible population. The distribution of live measles vaccine declined beginning with 1967. A reversal of the upward trend in measles cases noted in 1969 was reversed in 1972 coinciding with an increase in vaccine distribution beginning in 1971. Measles vaccine is more than 90 percent effective when given according to current recommendations. A review of the reasons for apparent vaccine failure leads to an estimate that two-thirds are the result of vaccinees who do not respond immunologically and the remaining one-third may be considered to have lost their immunity. Additional data suggest that immunity conferred with live measles vaccine is as effective as that after natural infection, and that two-thirds will have an immunity exceeding 10 years.

In assessing vaccination of children against rubella it is important to realize that the children receiving the vaccine are not the group which receive the major benefits. The principal health losses due to rubella are the congenital abnormalities which result from maternal infection early in pregnancy. An epidemic in 1964 and 1965, for example, resulted in 20,000 cases of congenital abnormalities attributed to rubella infection. However, since the safety of the vaccine has not been demonstrated in pregnant women, the transmission of the disease is controlled by vaccination of children. Epidemics of rubella occurred every six to nine years in the United States prior to the introduction of vaccine and thus an epidemic would have been expected in the early 1970s. The fact that it did not occur suggests that rubella vaccine used as a community protective agent is effective, but more complete evaluation of efficacy and length of immunity must await further observation.

It is fortunate that primary prevention of the above listed communicable diseases is feasible through vaccination of the target population and/or carriers of the disease. Unfortunately the system by which vaccinations are provided has not kept pace with development of immunologic agents. As noted in the case of measles, a resurgence of the disease followed a reduction in immunization levels and served as a reminder of the need for continuing immunization in the susceptible population. Declining immunization levels for poliomyelitis further emphasize the inadequacy of the current delivery system.

Manufacture of combined vaccines such as the measles-mumps-rubella vaccine helps in maintaining immunity to cover a larger number of diseases and susceptible groups, without an increase in personnel to administer the vaccine and inconvenience to the vaccinees. This is particularly important in the case of a disease such as mumps which is considered less of a public health problem than diseases such as measles or rubella. A combined vaccine may facilitate routine vaccination for mumps in the future. In combining several individual vaccines it is important to determine whether efficacy is reduced or adverse effects are increased. In the case of the measles-mumps-rubella vaccine it has been shown that the use of a combined vaccine provides a means for immunizing against the three diseases simultaneously, without any apparent reduction in efficacy and no significant increase in clinical reaction.

With the exception of smallpox, it is believed that the health gains and long-term beneficial effects greatly outweigh any detrimental effects associated with intervention in the form of immunization for the diseases listed earlier. It should be recognized that the nature of the threat of a particular disease may change so that future evaluation may not support continued application of the preventive procedure.

Screening for Hypertension

Hypertension is a condition of considerable magnitude. An estimated 23 million people can be classified as definite hypertensives (over 160 mm Hg systolic or 95 diastolic), about half of whom are in the age range 35–64. This is an important problem since hypertension is associated with increased risk for myocardial infarction, stroke, and other cardiovascular diseases. Approximately one and one quarter million excess deaths occur over a 10-year period in definite hypertensives age 35–64 when mortality rates of hypertensives are compared with those of normotensive persons. This same age group contains an additional 11 million persons who can be classified as borderline hypertensive (under 160/95 but over 140/95) with half a million excess deaths estimated. Fortunately high blood pressure is a condition which is easily identifiable. As a result there has been a considerable amount of effort devoted to determining the proper role of hypertension screening in preventive medicine and the efficacy of treatment in reducing hypertension and associated mortality due to cardiovascular disease.

The Veterans Administration Cooperative Study of Antihypertensive Agents provides firm evidence as to the effectiveness of detection and treatment in reducing mortality of patients with diastolic blood pressure averaging 115 through 129 mm Hg. A similar study of patients with blood pressure averaging 90 through 114 mm Hg resulted in mixed conclusions. Patients with diastolic blood pressure in the range of 90 to 104 mm Hg derived relatively little benefit from treatment unless they also had preexisting cardiovascular or renal complications or were over 50 years of age. It has been pointed out that the blood pressures recorded in the VA study were taken under basal or near basal conditions and at the "fifth phase" and thus the range 90–114 in the VA study may correspond to 110–124 in ordinary clinical practice. A further study is presently under way to determine whether pharmacological treatment of people with very mild hypertension (diastolic pressure 95 to 109 mm Hg) improves prognosis.

Since firm evidence does not exist to demonstrate the value of intervention in those with very mild hypertension, since patient compliance with a treatment regimen is frequently unsatisfactory, and because the cost effectiveness of mass screening may not equal or exceed the usual medical care available to patients with high blood pressure, several investigators have questioned whether extending mass screening for hypertension into the population at large is practical or justifiable at the present time. Additional work needs to be done in identifying risk factors which are useful in clearly identifying the most appropriate groups for screening, identifying persons with mild hypertension who may be at greatest risk, and whether and how much these persons with high risk will benefit from lowering of blood pressure. It is necessary to identify those who will progress to organic disease and treat them; the others receive little or no benefit from treatment. In the long run it appears obviously more desirable to control hypertension than to care for those who become disabled as a consequence of the disease. The exact levels of hypertension needing active treatment must be further defined. In the meantime the prudent course of action seems to be that guided by the Veterans Administration study, namely to treat many persons with hypertension at levels not previously regarded as requiring treatment.

Screening for Carcinoma of the Cervix

Cancer of the cervix uteri continues as a substantial health problem in the United States. In 1975 it is estimated that 7,800 deaths from the disease will occur.

Carcinoma-in-situ can be readily detected by an adequate cervical smear, although recognition must be given to false negatives depending on the quality of the cytology service. The natural history of the disease is much better understood than it was a quarter-century ago, but the exact risk of subsequent invasive disease associated with carcinoma-in-situ is not known. Evidence as to the effectiveness of cytology screening in reducing the incidence of invasive carcinoma of the cervix is still subject to doubt by some persons. However, various reports indicate that cytologic screening is correlated with a significant reduction of cancer incidence and mortality in areas with extensive screening. The extent to which this favorable trend can be attributed to cervical cancer screening is still questioned by some, but acceptance appears to be growing.

Participation in cervical screening has been shown to reach over 90% of the adult females in a population at least once, and most of them several times, when a program is continued for at least a decade. A realistic goal may be to screen almost the entire adult female population at least once every five to ten years. Since the in-situ stage may persist for this length of time before progressing to invasive disease this level of participation may be satisfactory as a community preventive measure. It should be noted, however, that those at highest risk for cervical carcinoma are least likely to present themselves for screening.

After evaluating the effectiveness of screening for cancer of the cervix, the Committee on Cancer Prevention and Detection of the International Union Against Cancer concluded that the use of cytology as a population screening procedure promises useful yields of preinvasive or early cancer and potential reduction in mortality.

The cost of detecting and treating a case of cervical carcinoma at the preclinical stage is less than the treatment of a clinical case; it is about half the cost. Thus screening for cervical cancer can be considered cost effective in the general population if it can be assumed that a majority of the cases with carcinoma-in-situ will progress to clinical disease.

On the basis of criteria set forth above as a means of evaluating preventive procedures, it is concluded that cervical cytology should be made available to the general adult female population.

Screening for Breast Cancer

With an estimated 88,000 new cases and 32,600 deaths in 1975, breast cancer is the leading cause of death from cancer in women. In the Health Insurance Plan population of New York City a controlled study offered women 40–64 years of age an annual breast cancer screening program with mammography and clinical examination of the breasts while a comparable group was kept as a control. It showed a reduction in mortality of one-third, even counting in the study group that portion (35 percent) who were offered the service but chose not to participate. The entire mortality reduction occurred among the women over 50 years of age; younger women did not appear to benefit. Both the clinical exam and mammography contributed independently to the detection of breast cancer; mammography was of particular importance in contributing to the mortality reduction. Although the efficacy of each screening procedure was not tested prior to combination, one analysis suggested that a significant proportion (over one-third) of the cancers would not have been detected if either procedure were used alone.

34

Although an effective screening procedure for breast cancer is available, the required number of trained professional and allied health personnel necessary to conduct a massive screening program involving major segments of the female population are not yet available. The National Cancer Institute/American Cancer Society breast cancer detection demonstration project in 27 centers and involving over one-quarter of a million women is addressing operational problems and probing into the results of screening in which palpation, mammography, and thermography are utilized. This study will provide data upon which the cost effectiveness of breast cancer screening can be better determined and improvements made.

At this time and with the techniques available, screening is relatively costly, particularly mammography. Until further research improves the cost effectiveness of breast cancer screening, provides for a clearer identification of age and other risk factors groups, and delineates better the risks of repeated radiation exposures, the expansion of breast cancer screening should be carried out on a selective basis. Questions that require further study are how often screening should be conducted and the lower age limit for offering routine screening. In the HIP study, the reduction in mortality was concentrated in the age group above 50; under 50 there was no reduction. Additional research on the age issue is needed.

Multiphasic Screening

Multiphasic screening refers to multiple tests given at the same time and aimed toward detection of various conditions that can be treated, as a means of improving health. This combining of tests is more economical and offers improved patient service compared with giving repeated batches of individual tests over an extended time period. Multiphasic screening helps redirect emphasis on preventive medicine and the provision of health maintenance to major segments of the population.

It is just as necessary in evaluating multiphasic screening as it is in evaluating individual preventive procedures that efficacy be measured in terms of end results. The periodic health examination utilizing automated multiphasic testing has been evaluated by investigation of changes in function and survival. Results showed that both function and survival were greater among the group encouraged to have multiphasic screening than among a control group.

Multiphasic screening procedures vary in content from a few tests to combinations involving a large battery of tests. Although there may be an overall efficacy shown for the entire battery, each individual test should be carefully evaluated to determine its contribution to the sum of the whole. Studies to further evaluate the effectiveness of multiphasic screening

35

programs of various types in improving function and survival are currently in progress.

It appears that over one-half of an appropriate population can be persuaded to participate in periodic multiphasic screening; a Kaiser Permanente study was successful in getting 65 percent of a study group to attend annually for a period of seven years. Acceptance by the medical profession has been slow. Multiphasic screening is viewed by many physicians as an intrusion into the patient-physician relationship. Only in prepayment group practice plans has multiphasic screening taken strong root.

The cost of multiphasic screening compares very favorably with the provision of the equivalent tests using traditional nonautomated methods. However, until costs are compared with evaluations of effectiveness or benefits it is not possible to judge if the gains measured in terms of end-results outweighs the financial cost and possible detrimental effects of intervention. A preliminary cost benefit analysis suggests that for a certain segment of the adult male population a small net saving results. In measuring the total cost associated with multiphasic screening it is important to include the cost of follow-up in asymptomatic screenees with positive test results. A significant amount of effort may be incurred in attempts at diagnosis and continued surveillance of asymptomatic patients.

Although at the present time periodic multiphasic screening cannot be recommended solely on the basis of cost effectiveness, it is the type of service increasingly made available to top executives of industry and high governmental officials.

While further detailed evaluations are pending, multiphasic health testing should be supported as one means of moving from crisis oriented medicine to that oriented toward health maintenance. To minimize the burden of false positive test results, multiphasic test packages should be tailored to specific population profiles, containing only tests which are appropriate and effective in the particular population.

Identification of Conditions and Procedures

A central issue in preventive medicine is the identification of preventive procedures that should be included as a standard part of personal health services. Each of the individual preventive medical procedures or tests that has been developed and applied successfully over the past years is an important element to be considered for the preventive medicine battery. However, if the application of preventive medicine is to become widespread in the general population a considerable amount of thought must be given to the particular conditions for which *effective* preventive procedures exist. It is desirable to identify a set of conditions and preventive procedures which could be recommended for application to the population at large, recognizing that certain special populations and high risk groups will always require additional preventive medicine beyond that required for the general population.

For a preventive medicine package to be appropriate and feasible for application to large segments of the general population it must include a "minimum" set of conditions and procedures, while at the same time being comprehensive enough to affect favorably the morbidity and mortality of the population. With this concept in mind, conditions and preventive procedures have been identified for various population age groups. Not all meet strictly the evaluation criteria listed earlier, generally because there is insufficient data available, not because of contrary evidence. A lack of conclusive supporting evidence in the absence of evidence to the contrary should not be interpreted as an indication that a particular procedure should not be applied. As noted earlier, prudence must be employed when scientific evidence is incomplete.

There is a minimum frequency with which any particular preventive package should be made available to the population if it is to be effective. For each of the sets of preventive procedures that are identified, a frequency is also stated in terms of the number of visits for each separate age group. The number of visits is considered to be the minimum that should be offered to the general population. If resources and finances permit, then the frequency could be increased.

Again it is important to recognize that high risk groups may require more frequent as well as additional procedures. Such an increase in risk may be due to a variety of genetic and environmental factors, including occupational hazards. In all cases, measures to prevent disease must be strategically used and based on population data. Strategies based on high risk are necessary to make optimum use of scarce resources. If we are to apply practical and cost efficient preventive programs to the entire population, high risk groups must be identified as a way to provide maximum benefit to the community as a whole. The latter does not necessarily provide maximum benefit to each individual regardless of cost.

Several approaches could be followed in devising a framework in which to recommend specific preventive procedures. A common approach and the one followed here is to segment the general population into age categories: mother and fetus; infant (newborn to 1 yr.); preschool child (1-6 yrs.); school age and adolescent (6-16 yrs.); young adult (17-34); middle-aged adult (35-64); older adult (65 yrs. and older). An alternative framework would have been to identify and categorize services by the groups which provide the service, for example, school health programs, private practice physicians, and public health departments.

The goals of preventive medicine for the mother and neonate should be:

1. To assure that the woman becomes pregnant on a planned basis and in a state of physical, mental, and social well-being; that this well-being is maintained throughout the pregnancy and postpartum period; that the mother has the knowledge and capacity to provide for the physical and emotional needs of the neonate.

2. To increase the likelihood that the pregnancy will proceed to term with a livebirth and the offspring will be normal (free of congenital or developmental damage).

To benefit the mother, the family, and the child, a preventive medicine program must start prior to the pregnancy: in school, at the time of marriage, and reinforced at critical points such as the postpartum period. Responses to deficiencies or problems detected will be heavily dependent on health education and counseling and appropriate follow-up. It should be noted that implications of 1. above include the right to abortion when there is a failure in family planning, and the mother, at an appropriately early stage of pregnancy, decides to terminate the pregnancy. The large reduction in maternal mortality that has accompanied the "right to abortion," by itself, is a justification for including abortion as a preventive health measure.

Preventive health services during the perinatal period are dependent on inventorying on a timely basis the great variety of background medical and social characteristics and intercurrent events that have been associated with poor perinatal outcome, to assess the need for altering the management of the pregnancy. Through a Committee on Perinatal Health—composed of representatives from the American Academy of Family Physicians, the American Academy of Pediatrics, the American College of Obstetricians and Gynecologists, and the American Medical Association and assisted by the National Foundation-March of Dimes—agreement is being reached among the professional organizations concerned with improving pregnancy outcome (i.e., reduction in mortality and morbidity among the newborn, particularly the sequelae of respiratory distress syndrome) on steps to be taken:

1. Risk assessment should start early in pregnancy and be maintained throughout pregnancy for new conditions.

2. Regionalization of perinatal care should provide for different levels of facilities and staffing for care of women (and in the immediate postpartum period, the neonate) with specified types of risks.

Provision should be made for an efficient graduation of specialized skills and facilities that optimizes the capacity within a health service region to respond to needs identified through risk assessment in 1. above. Included are opportunities for consultation and possible transfer of the high risk patient in a defined population. Based on limited experience in Canada and the U.S., the expectation is that not only will mortality be reduced but the surviving infant in a high risk pregnancy will less often be damaged and become a social and medical liability than is true among similar groups of infants today.

Table 3 lists the minimum conditions and preventive procedures directed toward the mother and fetus that should be included in a national health program.

The Infant

The goal of preventive medicine for the infant is to detect and treat certain diseases before damage occurs; to assure growth and development to the optimal potential of the child; and to provide for the prevention of specified infectious diseases through immunization.

Preventive procedures should be applied prior to discharge from the nursery and at four postdischarge visits up to one year of age. Prior to discharge the newborn should receive tests for inherited metabolic disorders which lead to mental retardation unless treated early, and for anemia, as well as observation and measurement for congenital malformations or disorders. After discharge the periodic visits should include observations and measurements directed toward growth and development disorders, including congenital malformations not previously detected, tests for iron deficiency anemia, immunizations, and parental counseling and education, as well as corrective medical care.

Table 4 identifies the procedures which are considered as the minimum to be included for adequate preventive care of the infant.

Preschool Child

The basic conditions of interest in this age group are growth and development. Observations should occur at least twice, once at age two to three and again at age five to six. Development observation includes nutrition, vision, hearing, speech, dental health, and mental, behavioral, and general physical development. Assuming that primary immunization in the first year has included at least DTP and TOPV, the second year adds measles, mumps, and rubella. The preschool exam repeats DTP and TOPV. Hemoglobin determination at two years and school entry is the only universal laboratory screen recommended. Conditions such as lead poisoning and tuberculin sensitivity are highly important, but for special groups only.

Table 3: Mother and Fetus

PROCEDURE	CONDITION	TYPE OF PREVENTION	INTERVENTION
History of menarche	Unplanned pregnancy (before pregnancy)	1	Contraception
Serological Exam	Lack of Rubella antibody (before pregnancy)	1	Immunization
Pregnancy Test	Unwanted pregnancy	2	Abortion
History of pregnancy	Unsuccessful prior pregnancy	2	Counseling
History and Counseling	Inadequate preparation for pregnancy	1	Counseling
History and Counseling	Inadequate preparation for delivery	1	Counseling
History and Counseling	Inadequate preparation for parenthood	1	Counseling
History and Counseling	Smoking and other risks to developing fetus	1, 2	Counseling
History and Counseling	Inadequate recognition of signs and symptoms of abnormalities	1	Counseling
Anthropometric Examination and Counseling	Nutritional abnormality	2	Counseling and Diet
Hemoglobin/Hematocrit	Anemia	2	Diagnosis and therapy
Urine albumen	Toxemia	2	Diagnosis and therapy
Pap smear	Genital tract malignancy	2	Diagnosis and therapy
VDRL	Syphilis	2	Diagnosis and therapy Counseling and contact finding
G. C. culture	Gonorrhea	2	Penicillin, Counseling and contact finding
Blood grouping and Rh determination	Rh iso-immunization and other blood abnormalities	1	Antibody
Casual blood sugar	Abnormal glucose tolerance	2	Diagnosis and therapy
Blood pressure measurement	Hypertension	2	Diagnosis and therapy
Examination	Organic heart disease	2	Diagnosis and therapy
Physical Exam	Pelvic inadequacy	2	Diagnosis and therapy
Physical Exam	Reproductive organ abnormality	2	Diagnosis and therapy
Urine culture	Bacteriuria (after third pregnancy)	2	Diagnosis and therapy
Amniocentesis	Genetic disorders (women over age 40)	2	Diagnosis and therapy
Blood Test	Sickle Cell trait (High risk groups only)	2	Diagnosis and therapy

Table 4. Infant[a]

PROCEDURE	CONDITION	TYPE OF PREVENTION	INTERVENTION
History and Counseling	Inadequate preparation for infant care (newborn)	1	Parent Counseling
PKU	Metabolic disorders (newborn)	2	Diagnosis and therapy
Silver nitrate prophylaxis	Gonorrheal ophthalmia (newborn)	1	Prophylaxis
Observation and measurement	Congenital malformations (newborn)	2	Diagnosis and therapy
Vaccinations	Diphtheria, Tetanus and Pertussis	1	Immunization
TOPV	Poliomyelitis	1	Immunization
Vitamin K	Hemorrhagic disease	1	Prophylaxis
Hematocrit	Anemia	2	Diagnosis and therapy
Developmental assessment including height and weight	Growth and development disorders	2	Diagnosis and therapy
Counseling	Accidents	1	Parent Counseling

[a]Newborn plus four visits after discharge

Preventive counseling of mothers should cover a wide gamut of matters, but especially nutrition and hygiene (including dental), compliance with immunization protocol, and prevention of accidents and poisoning. A universal counseling need is behavioral in its broadest sense. The huge distribution of books such as that by Spock indicates the need of mothers for guidance. Many later problems may reflect lack of, or improper, counseling of mothers with children in this age group.

Table 5 lists the preventive procedures for the one-to-six-year age group. While this is a very simple list, it is difficult to justify any additional preventive procedure that is generally needed for all children at this, fortunately, relatively healthy age. The low use of hospital services for this age group reflects the good health of preschool children in the United States; hospital use would be even less if nonrational therapy such as many tonsillectomies were avoided.

School Age and Adolescent

During school age, mortality rates reach their lowest level. The 1975 U.S. life tables show that only 0.38 percent of those alive at age five die before they reach the age of 15 years. Nonetheless, these years are of importance, perhaps second only to the preschool years, in establishing the foundations which determine future good or ill health.

During this period a minimum of two health supervision visits (for healthy children) are indicated, with at least one of these visits including a

Table 5. Age 1–6 Years[a]

PROCEDURE	CONDITION	TYPE OF PREVENTION	INTERVENTION
Observation and assessments	Growth and development abnormalities	2	Diagnosis and therapy
Observation and assessments	Neurologic disorders	2	Diagnosis and therapy
Anthropometric measurements	Malnutrition and obesity	1, 2	Counseling and diet
Hematocrit	Anemia	2	Diagnosis and therapy
Hearing and vision testing	Hearing, vision, and eye deficiencies	2	Diagnosis and therapy
Speech testing	Communication disorders	2	Diagnosis and therapy
Vaccination	Diphtheria, Tetanus, and Pertussis	1	Immunization
History and vaccination if indicated	Measles, Mumps, and Rubella	1	Immunization
History and TOPV if indicated	Poliomyelitis	1	Immunization
Dental exam	Dental defects	1, 2	Diagnosis and therapy
Counseling	Accidents	1	Parent Counseling
Counseling	Poisoning	1	Parent Counseling

[a]One visit at age two to three and one at age five to six.

physical examination done by a physician or by an appropriately trained physician-assistant. One visit should occur at age 8–9 and one at age 13–14. During both these visits a complete medical history should be obtained with a history of cigarette smoking and the use of drugs or alcohol on the second visit.

Advantage should be taken of the early adolescent opportunity to provide counseling and education with particular reference to accident prevention and sex problems including the use of contraceptives.

If there are gaps in the immunization record, with particular reference to rubella and mumps, these should be corrected. If rubella vaccine is given in the later years, precautions should be taken to insure that female vaccinees do not become pregnant during the succeeding months. The second visit should include immunization for diphtheria and tetanus.

Minimal testing for this age group includes:

1. Measurement of height and weight to identify possible malnutrition and obesity.
2. Visual acuity among children ages 6 to 11 years, since 11 percent have poor distance vision and 6 percent poor near vision. Among children aged 12 to 17 years, the corresponding figures are 22 percent for distance vision and 9 percent for near vision.
3. Hearing. About 1 percent of school children have a significant

hearing loss. Such hearing loss can account for problems in both language and learning.

4. Several easy tests for ascertaining intellectual ability and physical coordination, appropriate for each age group, can be used to identify significant learning disability or muscular incoordination. Problems of this nature can be a serious handicap, as can significant speech problems.

5. Abnormal blood pressure values are uncommon during primary school life but a few surgically amenable conditions do occur which will benefit from early diagnosis.

6. Towards the end of school life at least one blood specimen should be taken for hemoglobin determination. Low hemoglobin values frequently have little significance by themselves but may suggest a general state of malnutrition or anemia which needs attention.

7. Among selected high risk populations there may be indication for additional tests including urine examination for sugar, albumen, and bacteria (among girls); sickle cell testing; and for young girls who are sexually active, pregnancy testing, GC screening, and VDRL.

These and additional preventive procedures relating to dental health, acne, and counseling, particularly on accident prevention, are summarized in Table 6.

Young Adult

Table 7 lists the minimum conditions and preventive procedures that should be provided to all young adults through the personal health services sysem. Three visits should take place during the 17–35 age period: one at 17 or 18 years of age, one at about age 25 and the other at about age 30.

The minimum battery of preventive measures includes some procedures which can be recommended on the basis of conclusive evidence that improvement in mortality or morbidity results from intervention, such as immunization booster against tetanus and diphtheria, VDRL and GC culture for prevention of tertiary syphilis and symptomatic gonorrhea, and the diagnosis and treatment of malnutrition. Several other procedures are included on the basis of indirect evidence or on the basis of prudence. The effectiveness of treatment for mild degrees of hypertension in the young adult has not been finally established. However, prudence based on the proven efficacy of intervention at a later age strongly supports blood pressure measurement and treatment of mild as well as severe degrees of hypertension as an important preventive procedure in

Table 6. Age 6–16 Years[a]

PROCEDURE	CONDITION	TYPE OF PREVENTION	INTERVENTION
Observation and assessment	Behavioral, intellectual, or communicative maladjustments	2	Counseling Diagnosis and therapy
History and counseling	Smoking	1, 2	Counseling
Examination and prophylaxis	Dental caries Malocclusions Periodontal disease	1, 2	Prophylaxis Diagnosis and therapy
Hearing and vision testing	Visual and hearing defects	2	Diagnosis and therapy
Anthropometric examination	Musculoskeletal disorders	2	Diagnosis and therapy
Anthropometric examination	Malnutrition including underweight or overweight	1, 2	Counseling and diet
Skin examination	Acne	2	Diagnosis and treatment
History and examination	Sexual immaturity or disorders (2nd visit only)	1, 2	Counseling Diagnosis and therapy
Counseling	Accidents	1	Counseling
Vaccination	Diphtheria Tetanus (2nd visit only)	1	Immunization boosters
History	Drug abuse and alcohol (2nd visit only)	1, 2	Counseling
Hematocrit	Anemia (2nd visit only)	2	Diagnosis and treatment
Blood pressure	Cardiovascular problems (2nd visit only)	2	Diagnosis and treatment
History	Unwanted pregnancy (2nd visit for high risk groups only)	1	Contraception
VDRL	Syphilis (2nd visit for high risk groups only)	2	Diagnosis and treatment Counseling and contact finding
G.C. Culture	Gonorrhea (2nd visit for high risk groups only)	2	Diagnosis and treatment Counseling and contact finding

[a]One visit at age 8–9 and one at age 13–14.

the young adult. Hematocrit and cholesterol testing are also included on the basis of prudence, even though conclusive evidence for the efficacy of treating mild degrees of asymptomatic anemia is lacking, and a change in diet to reduce an elevated cholesterol level can be supported only as a potential means of decreasing the risk of coronary artery disease. Similarly the inclusion of screening for cervical cancer and especially for breast cancer in young females is based on reasonable interpretation of available data. Only in older adults does firm evidence exist for breast cancer screening. Cessation of cigarette smoking does reduce the risk of heart and lung disease, and the use of seat belts and not driving while under the influence of alcohol reduces both the number and the consequences of automobile accidents. Thus counseling as a means of favorably influencing these conditions is included in the recommended list of preventive procedures.

Middle-Aged Adult

Table 8 summarizes the preventive procedures that are considered minimal for the 35 to 64 year age group. At least one visit every five years beginning at age 35 and ending at age 60 is considered necessary. Those persons above 64 years of age are included in the older adult group.

Middle-aged adults should receive preventive services beyond those provided to the young adult group. A stool guaiac should be included as a screen for cancer (further studies of efficacy are in progress) and a glucose test for diabetes. For a positive glucose tolerance test, without other

Table 7.   Ages 17–34[a]

PROCEDURE	CONDITION	TYPE OF PREVENTION	INTERVENTION
History of completed immunization or booster in past 10 years	Tetanus Diphtheria	1	Td Vaccine
Rubella HI	Congenital Rubella Syndrome (females only)	1	Rubella Vaccine
VDRL	Syphilis	2	Diagnosis and Treatment
GC Culture of Female	Gonorrhea	2	Diagnosis and Treatment; Contact Investigation
Height and Weight	Malnutrition and Obesity	1, 2	Counseling and Diet Diagnosis-Treatment
Blood Pressure	Hypertension and Associated Conditions and Complications	1, 2	Diagnosis and Treatment
Cholesterol	Coronary Artery Disease	1	Counseling and Diet
Hematocrit	Anemia	2	Diagnosis and Treatment
Casual Blood Sugar	Abnormal Glucose Tolerance and Diabetes	1, 2	Diagnosis and Treatment
Cervical Cytology	Cancer of Cervix	2	Diagnosis and Treatment
Breast Exam (self)	Breast Cancer	2	Diagnosis and Treatment
Hearing and Vision Testing	Hearing and Visual Acuity Disorders	2	Diagnosis and Treatment
History/Life Style	Heart and Lung Diseases	1, 2	Counseling
History and Counseling	Alcoholism and Drugs	1, 2	Counseling
Counseling	Accidents	2	Counseling
History and Counseling	Smoking	1, 2	Counseling
PPD	Tuberculosis (high risk groups only)	2	Diagnosis and Treatment

[a] One visit at ages 17–18, 25, and 30.

Table 8. Age 35–64[a]

PROCEDURE	CONDITION	TYPE OF PREVENTION	INTERVENTION
History of completed immunization or booster in past 10 years	Tetanus Diphtheria	1	Td Vaccine
VDRL	Syphilis	2	Diagnosis and Treatment
Height and Weight	Malnutrition and Obesity	1, 2	Counseling and Diet Diagnosis Treatment
Blood Pressure	Hypertension and Associated Conditions and Complications	1, 2	Diagnosis and Treatment
Cholesterol	Coronary Artery Disease	1	Counseling and Diet
Hematocrit	Anemia	2	Diagnosis and Treatment
Stool for blood	Occult malignancy	2	Diagnosis and Treatment
Glucose Tolerance Test	Diabetes	2	Diagnosis and Treatment
Breast exam	Breast Cancer	2	Diagnosis and Treatment
Mammography or Xerography in all over age 50, and high risk less than age 50	Breast Cancer (more frequent than every five years)	2	Diagnosis and Treatment
History/Life Style	Heart and Lung Disease	1, 2	Counseling
Hearing and Vision Testing	Hearing and Vision Disorders	2	Diagnosis and Treatment
History and Counseling	Alcoholism and Drugs	1, 2	Counseling
History and Counseling	Smoking	1, 2	Counseling
Counseling	Accidents	1	Counseling
Cervical Smear	Cervix Cancer	2	Diagnosis and Treatment
PPD	Tuberculosis (high risk groups only)	2	Diagnosis and Treatment

[a] One visit every five years from age 40 to 60.

evidence of diabetes, counseling about diet is the choice of intervention; unnecessary drug treatment should be avoided. The efficacy of mammography in combination with breast examination has been well established (at least over the short term) in women over 50 years of age. However, on the basis of existing evidence the test should be administered more frequently than every five years.

Many other specific measures were considered but excluded from this set. Some were not included after noting that if a particular abnormality or condition is found in an asymptomatic individual there is little evidence that intervention at that point would be of any value. For example, there is no evidence that tonometry detects the condition at a time when the natural history of the disease can be changed, i.e., there is no evidence that their experience is any different from individuals detected and treated when they first get symptoms. In this case, however, secondary screening for peripheral vision of those found to have elevated intraocular tension is being studied to ascertain its value in avoiding the adverse effects of glaucoma before symptoms are noted.

Older Adult

Table 9 lists preventive procedures for the population aged 65 or over. A visit is considered necessary every two years. Procedures to be added for this age group include influenza immunization for protection of the elderly who are at high risk for complications of influenza, and on the basis of indirect evidence EKG is included for detection of cardiac arrhythmia. Although the prevalence of glaucoma is high in this age group, tonometry is again not included as a routine procedure because of lack of sufficient evidence as to the effectiveness of treatment.

Counseling as it relates to preparation for retirement and the associated change in life style is also included as a prudent procedure for this age group.

Table 9.   Age 65 or Over[a]

PROCEDURE	CONDITION	TYPE OF PREVENTION	INTERVENTION
History of completed immunization or booster in past 10 years	Tetanus Diphtheria	1	Td Vaccine
Influenza immunization	Influenza and Complications	1	Influenza Vaccine
Height and Weight	Malnutrition and Obesity	1, 2	Counseling and Diet Diagnosis-Treatment
Blood Pressure	Hypertension and Associated Conditions and Complications	1, 2	Diagnosis and Treatment
EKG	Arrhythmia	2	Diagnosis and Treatment
Hearing and Vision Testing	Hearing and Vision Deficiencies	2	Diagnosis and Treatment
Glucose Tolerance Test	Diabetes	2	Diagnosis and Treatment
Hematocrit	Anemia	2	Diagnosis and Treatment
Stool for Blood	Occult GI Disease	2	Diagnosis and Treatment
Breast Exam and Mammography or Xerography	Breast Cancer	2	Diagnosis and Treatment
History/Life Style	Heart and Lung Disease	1, 2	Counseling
History and Counseling	Alcoholism and Drugs	1, 2	Counseling
History and Counseling	Depression and Suicide	1, 2	Counseling
Counseling	Accidents	1	Counseling

[a] One visit every two years

47

Justification of Concerted Effort

An important issue in preventive medicine is whether the time is at hand for a concerted effort to incorporate such packages of preventive medical procedures systematically into personal health services.

Does the totality of conditions for which preventive procedures can be applied effectively justify including preventive medicine as a major thrust in personal health services? There can be little debate on the subject of whether certain preventive procedures should be included as part of the health service system, particularly the various immunizations. However, the point being raised here is whether a sufficient number of useful preventive procedures are available to justify their systematic routine incorporation into the personal health service system. Is the potential of preventive medicine as defined in this report now great enough to call for a fundamental change in the health service system, a change that would make preventive medicine an organizing and guiding element in personal health service rather than a minor and occasional appendage in a system mainly geared for episodic care? Should the system focus be made health maintenance rather than complaint response?

Several expert, professional groups have during the past three years prepared "packages" of recommended preventive medical procedures. Three such packages proposed for inclusion in National Health Insurance are presented in Appendix II. These packages have been developed on behalf of the American Public Health Association, the Association of Schools of Public Health and the Association of Teachers of Preventive Medicine, and the Fogarty International Center.

It is of interest to see how these other three packages compare with the minimum list of preventive procedures presented in this Task Force report. Tables 10 to 16 show this comparison. It should be noted that it was necessary to make certain judgments since the age categories used for the different packages did not correspond exactly. Furthermore various tests may have been implied which were not explicitly identified. For example, the APHA package mentioned only that laboratory examination should be carried out for children without specifying the specific tests. Certain procedures such as height and weight determination have been assumed to be included in the physical exam.

Although it is clear that some differences exist among the "packages" of preventive medicine procedures set forth by the four professional groups, these differences are very minor compared with the similarities of the proposals. The principal differences are that one group (FIC) called for a somewhat more extensive list of procedures than did the other three. The latter differed only mildly in detail. The principal similarities are these:

Table 10. Mother and Fetus

	FIC[a]	ASPH, ATPM[b]	APHA[c]	TF[d]
History (includes previous pregnancy)	X	X	X	X
Height and Weight	X	X	X	X
Blood Pressure	X	X	X	X
Temperature	X			
Physical Examination	X	X	X	X
Dental Examination	X			
Laboratory Examinations				
Hemoglobin/Hematocrit	X	X	X	X
Blood Count, complete			X	
Blood Smear	X			
Rubella Antibody	X			X
Au Antigen	X			
Rh Determination (mother and father)	X	X	X	X
Blood Grouping	X	X	X	X
Biochemical Profile	X			
Blood Sugar				X
Urinalysis, complete	X		X	
Urine-Sugar and Albumen		X		X
VDRL	X	X	X	X
Tuberculin	X			
Gonococcal Culture	X		X	X
Pap Smear	X		X	X
Chest x-ray			X	
Tetanus Immunization	X			
Counseling				
Family Planning	X		X	
Nutrition	X	X	X	X
Smoking	X	X		X
Disorders of Early Pregnancy	X			X
Risks to Developing Fetus	X			X
Abortion	X			
Congenital Anomalies	X			
Labor and Delivery	X	X	X	X
Infant Care	X		X	
Parenthood			X	X
Self Care			X	X
Additional Procedures for Certain Groups				
Cephalometry	X			
Tachodynamometry	X			
Urine Culture	X			X
Urinary Estrogen/Creatinine	X			
Urinary Urea N/Total N	X			
Amniocentesis	X			X
Gamma Globulin	X			
Anti-Rh Titers	X			

[a]Preventive medical services for National Health Insurance. Report of a Fogarty International Center Task Force prepared under the auspices of the Office of the Assistant Secretary for Health, DHEW, May 1974.

[b]Incorporation of preventive medical services into National Health Insurance. A paper prepared for the Office of Management and Budget by Lester Breslow on behalf of the Association of Schools of Public Health and the Association of Teachers of Preventive Medicine, November 19, 1973.

[c]Proposed preventive benefits to be covered on a first-dollar-basis under National Health Insurance. The American Public Health Association, July 16, 1974.

[d]The preventive procedures proposed in this task force report.

Table 11. Infant

	FIC	ASPH, ATPM	APHA	TF
Height and Weight	X	X	X	X
Head Circumference	X			
Vision and Hearing	X			
Physical Examination	X	X	X	X
Development Assessment	X	X	X	X
PKU	X	X		X
Serological Testing			X	X
Hematocrit	X			X
Tuberculin	X			
Silver Nitrate Prophylaxis				X
Vitamin K				X
DTP Vaccination	X	X	X	X
TOPV	X	X	X	X
Counseling of Parents				
Nutrition	X	X	X	
Infant Care (includes hygiene and feeding)	X	X	X	X
Accidents	X	X	X	X
Poisons	X			
Infant Behavior		X		

Table 12. Preschool Child

	FIC	ASPH, ATPM	APHA	TF
Height and Weight	X	X	X	X
Blood Pressure	X			
Vision and Hearing	X	X	X	X
Speech	X	X		X
Physical Examination	X	X	X	X
Dental Examination	X	X	X	X
Development and Behavior Assessment	X	X	X	X
Hematocrit	X			
Urinalysis	X	X		
Urine Culture (females)	X	X		
Tuberculin	X			
DTP Vaccination	X	X	X	X
TOPV	X	X	X	X
Measles-Mumps-Rubella	X	X	X	X
Parent and Child Counseling				
Nutrition	X	X	X	
Oral Hygiene	X		X	
Smoking	X			
Accidents		X	X	X
Poisons				X

Table 13.   Schoolchild and Adolescent

	FIC	ASPH, ATPM	APHA	TF
Height and Weight	X	X	X	X
Blood Pressure	X	X		X
Vision and Hearing	X	X	X	X
Physical Examination (including skin)	X	X	X	X
Dental Examination	X	X	X	X
Development Assessment	X	X	X	X
Laboratory Examinations				
Cholesterol	X	X		
Hematocrit	X			
Urinalysis		X		X
Urine Culture (females)	X	X		
VDRL	X	X		
Tuberculin	X			X
Sickle Cell Trait	X			
Gonococcal Culture (females)	X	X		X
Immunization Boosters	X	X	X	X
Counseling				
Nutrition	X	X		
Oral Hygiene	X			
Smoking	X	X		X
Drugs	X	X	X	X
Alcohol	X	X	X	X
Sexual Development and Hygiene	X	X	X	X
Family Planning and Contraception	X	X		X
Exercise		X		
Accidents	X	X		X

1. All of them listed definite preventive procedures for specific age groups, instead of calling for a vague "check-up."

2. All of them indicated some rational periodicity, rather than an annual "check-up."

3. All of them relied both on scientific proof and on prudent interpretation of all available evidence concerning potential benefits and costs.

4. All of them included both certain counseling procedures designed to influence favorably habits related to health (such as cigarette smoking), and certain physical procedures designed to ascertain such health risk indicators as blood pressure and blood cholesterol as a basis for preventive medical action.

5. All of them agreed fully on many of the specific procedures, and there was substantial agreement (three out of four) on several more. A good number of the apparent discrepancies were undoubtedly due to coding problems, for example, the failure to include for the preschool child counseling on nutrition by the present Task Force, and on accidents by the FIC group.

It is remarkable that within a three-year period, four separate

Table 14.   Young Adult

	FIC	ASPH, ATPM	APHA	TF
History	X		X	X
Height and Weight	X	X	X	X
Blood Pressure	X	X		X
EKG	X			
Hearing and Vision				X
Physical Examination	X	X	X	X
Breast Examination (females)			X	X
Rectal Examination			X	
Pelvic Examination (females)			X	
Laboratory Examinations				
Cholesterol	X	X		X
Triglycerides	X			
Glucose/Blood Sugar	X			X
Uric Acid	X			
SGOT	X			
Hemoglobin/Hematocrit	X			X
Blood Count, complete			X	
Urinalysis	X	X	X	
VDRL			X	X
Gonococcal Culture (females)		X	X	X
Pap Smear (females)	X	X	X	X
Chest x-ray			X	
Tetanus and Diphtheria Boosters	X			X
Counseling				
Nutrition		X	X	
Smoking	X	X	X	X
Alcohol and Drugs	X	X		X
Contraception and Family Planning			X	
Exercise		X	X	
Sleep		X		
Accidents				X

professional bodies, expert in preventive medicine and public health, have presented such similar recommendations: the Association of Schools of Public Health and the Association of Teachers of Preventive Medicine; the American Public Health Association; a task force assembled by the Fogarty International Center of the National Institutes of Health; and a National Conference on Preventive Medicine sponsored by the American College of Preventive Medicine and the Fogarty International Center of the National Institutes of Health. While there was, as might be expected from the nature of the field, some overlap of personnel involved, it is clear that the composite proposal emerging represents a very high degree of concurrence among the nation's experts in preventive medicine and public health.

Agreement on a final list of age groups and procedures could probably be reached by representatives of the four groups within a few days, if that should prove desirable.

Implementation of Preventive Medicine

In considering the various issues surrounding the theory and application of preventive medicine in personal health services, it is important that recognition be given to the state of health service system readiness to provide preventive care. It is clear that the personal health service system needs to be tuned for that purpose. Before large-scale introduction of even a single preventive procedure, attention must be given to system readiness.

Also, each procedure needs to be continually reviewed and evaluated on the basis of new information concerning efficacy, adverse effects, and

Table 15.   Middle Age Adult

	FIC	ASPH, ATPM	APHA	TF
History	X		X	X
Height and Weight	X		X	X
Blood Pressure	X	X	X	X
EKG	X	X	X	
Vision		X	X	
Tonometry	X	X		X
Spirometry			X	
Physical Examination	X	X	X	
Breast Examination (females)		X	X	X
Rectal Examination		X	X	
Sigmoidoscopy			X	
Pelvic Examination (females)			X	
Laboratory Examinations				
Cholesterol	X	X	X	X
Triglycerides	X		X	
Glucose/Blood Sugar	X	X		X
Uric Acid	X			
SGOT	X			
Hemoglobin/Hematocrit	X			X
Blood Count, complete			X	
BUN			X	
Creatinine			X	
Urinalysis	X		X	
VDRL			X	
Tuberculin			X	X
Gonococcal Culture (females)			X	
Pap Smear (females)	X	X	X	X
Stool Guaiac	X	X	X	X
Mammography (females)	X	X		X
Chest x-ray			X	
Tetanus and Diphtheria Boosters	X			X
Counseling				
Nutrition		X	X	
Smoking	X	X	X	X
Alcohol and Drugs	X	X		X
Contraception			X	
Exercise		X	X	
Sleep		X		
Accidents				X

Table 16. Older Adult

	FIC	ASPH, ATPM	APHA	TF
History	X		X	X
Height and Weight	X	X	X	X
Blood Pressure	X	X	X	X
EKG	X	X	X	X
Vision	X	X		X
Tonometry		X	X	
Hearing	X	X		X
Spirometry			X	
Physical Examination	X	X	X	X
Breast Examination (females)	X			X
Rectal Examination	X	X	X	
Sigmoidoscopy			X	
Podiatric Examination	X			
Dental Examination	X			
Laboratory Examinations				
Cholesterol	X		X	
Triglycerides	X		X	
Glucose/Blood Sugar	X	X		X
Uric Acid	X			
SGOT	X			
Hemoglobin/Hematocrit	X			X
Blood Count, complete			X	
BUN			X	
Creatinine			X	
Urinalysis	X		X	
VDRL			X	
Tuberculin			X	
Pap Smear (females)	X	X		X
Stool Guaiac	X	X	X	X
Mammography (females)		X		X
Chest x-ray			X	
Tetanus and Diphtheria Boosters	X			X
Influenza Immunization	X			X
Counseling				
Nutrition	X	X	X	
Smoking	X		X	
Alcohol and Drugs	X	X		X
Social Habits	X			
Exercise		X	X	
Sleep		X		
Housing	X			
Retirement Plans		X		
Depression/Suicide				X
Accidents				X

costs. Perhaps a federally supported commission should be established to carry out continuing evaluation of this nature. Such a commission could provide a focus for and coordinate existing evaluation efforts now being carried out in various bureaus of the Federal Government; unnecessary duplication should be avoided. The impact of any proposed governmental regulation in preventive medicine should be studied. A certain amount of regulation may be needed, particularly when health risks are involved as in radiographic procedures, or when significant resources are involved as in the implementation of computer-assisted transaxial tomography. Units for the latter are being approved for installation only after a review of factors beyond efficacy, such as need and geographic distribution. A review of this nature helps assure that, because of limitations on financial resources, one capability is not unnecessarily developed to the displacement of some other capability.

Another important issue in the implementation of preventive medicine is that the appropriate population groups are addressed. There may be a tendency to focus personal health services on the older age groups since it is during this period of life that many of the conditions and diseases strike. However, particularly for prevention, that stage is often too late for optimal effectiveness. We need to target much of our effort in an earlier age group.

For preventive medicine to achieve its greatest potential it is necessary to give special emphasis to high risk groups. More attention, for example, should be given to groups that have had special exposure to cancer-causing agents. Special financial resources should be provided for reaching high risk groups within a population; merely drawing attention to this need is not enough. However, risk is not a yes-no situation, and it is frequently difficult to identify high risk groups with great precision. The strategy, of course, is intended to allow recruitment of the most susceptible populations into particular preventive medicine programs and to discourage others from overutilization of services.

Overutilization can become a problem in preventive medicine as it has in other areas of medicine. If a preventive procedure is established as a part of personal health services, then it is difficult to discourage people from using it, sometimes to excess. For example, annual chest x-ray examinations have been performed on many people in this country with dubious justification.

A limited amount of data is available which indicates that, given uninhibited access, utilization of preventive services is high in groups that need preventive medicine. There is a greater use of preventive services, for example, by subscribers to group practice prepayment plans than individuals with other health insurance plans or no plan at all.

Legislation is another way to influence utilization of preventive services. Further work needs to be done on determining the extent to which laws can be helpful or hinder in the application of preventive medicine. States are taking legislative action favoring use of preventive services, which provides opportunity for observing its influence on patterns of use.

Prudence requires that adverse side effects and other costs are weighed against benefits in the decision to move ahead in the expansion of preventive medicine. As an example, multiphasic screening should expand only in the light of explicit and careful consideration to the effectiveness and cost of follow-up. The latter, for example, may result in services to some people with positive test results but no condition that justifies treatment. That must be placed in balance with those who benefit. Similarly, the long-term effects of pharmaceutical materials and the possibility of iatrogenic disease needs to be considered. This caution is particularly cogent in the consideration of new technological advancements. Without extensive studies, risks associated with the utilization of a new technique or procedure may not be known. The potential risk associated with tomography is a current topic of discussion and investigation.

It is clear that a variety of socioeconomic factors have a direct influence on the implementation of preventive medicine. The specific preventive procedures which are available for application, the readiness of the personal health services system, the utilization by the population and the associated costs and medical risks all affect implementation.

Organization and Financing

Another major influence, and one perhaps of greatest influence on implementation, is the way in which preventive services are organized and the financial arrangements that affect access.

It is necessary to identify forms of organization of personal health service delivery that will be most effective for the provision of preventive medicine. Traditionally, an organization to provide care is set up and then an assessment to determine whether it is accomplishing its goals may follow. Resources to continue this sequential approach are not plentiful. It is becoming desirable to assess the potential effectiveness of proposed organizational designs before implementation.

An important issue in how one organizes for preventive medicine is the extent to which different ways of providing it to the public can be used. Various preventive packages are offered in various settings. It is necessary to determine what is best done in campaigns, industry, special populations, school settings, or other situations. Different procedures may be carried out in different programs. Some new preventive procedures may best be carried out in a campaign rather than waiting for the procedure to filter into the community. Commonly a procedure is developed; tested in clinical situations, for example, medical centers; evaluated with an imperfect design on some community groups; adopted by a few "enthusiasts," and gradually spreads in use. Sometimes this process takes years. Occasionally a procedure which meets all reasonable criteria is suitable for a large proportion of the population, but is not applied systematically. In fact, after an ambitious initial campaign has achieved its goal, it may be difficult to sustain a satisfactory level of application. For example, the initial poliomyelitis and measles campaigns were very successful but in recent years the level of immunization in some communities has dropped to levels which again permit epidemic outbreaks.

The groups and settings established to further the application of preventive medicine should be of sufficient size and nature that organizational structures of reasonable scope can be built up. For maximum long-term effect, the organization of preventive services should involve a variety of providers in totality offering a full spectrum of preventive services to all persons, with an adequate follow-up.

No single type of health professional exists that is ideally suited to provide the full spectrum of preventive services. A team or cadre of health professionals is needed in the implementation of a comprehensive preventive program, with each member serving in the role for which he or she is best suited. Education and training are needed to make this team or any other organized approach to preventive medicine work. Specialized preventive medicine experts, allied health personnel, and the family physician all need to be trained in an integrative approach to the implementation of preventive medicine in personal health services.

An organizational setting should be provided so that counseling, motivation, education, screening, and other preventive services are all tied together.

Until a particular level of activity is reached it may not be cost effective to provide certain counseling services. Without the involvement of physicians generally in the community there may be inadequate follow-up for those needing therapy. It may cost more to provide preventive service in a particular setting but improved follow-up and linkage with traditional medicine may offset this additional cost.

An optimal organization framework for preventive medicine also entails checks to insure that everyone is within the system. Without this check the very population subgroups that most need preventive medicine service may not receive it.

One approach to overcoming this potential problem is to identify specific populations for which various provider groups are responsible. This responsibility should include adequate follow-up. When intervention beyond primary or secondary prevention is required, the patients' transition into the tertiary component of the health care system should be assured. The provision of preventive, diagnostic, therapeutic, and continuing care should be viewed as a continuum.

It is also necessary to determine what forms of payment and financing are most effective for inclusion of preventive medicine in personal health services. Unified financing of all personal health services is, in general, desirable to facilitate a comprehensive and unified approach to the provision of health services including preventive services. However, to insure that preventive medicine gets an adequate share of financial support it may be necessary to require a specified portion of funding for prevention.

It is important that preventive medicine not continue to suffer as a "poor relation," fiscally, of traditional episodic medicine.

Preventive medicine should receive at least as high priority for financial support as episodic medicine. Reimbursement should be provided for at least a minimum preventive package. Preventive services must be treated the same as therapeutic services in any type of prepayment or national health insurance program that is finally adopted.

Without full reimbursement there will be a truncation of preventive services. For example, one study has clearly shown that the amount of preventive medicine delivered to a population is substantially lower if copayment is required than if it is not required. This effect of copayment should be clearly realized and not permitted for those specific preventive medicine procedures that should receive widespread application. Furthermore, special high risk groups identified on the basis of demographic and biological characteristics should receive additional financial support for special entitlements.

Research

Scientific and technical advance is a fundamental force in the expansion of preventive medicine in personal health services. Actually having the means to prevent disease constitutes the main thrust to their application. Hence, research and development seeking more effective means of disease prevention is essential to realizing the full potential of the field. In addition to encouragement of epidemiology per se, particularly for identifying high risk groups, it is desirable to expand collaboration with those in physiology, immunology, and the other basic science fields in which fundamental progress may yield new clues to disease control.

Research and development are also needed to translate existing knowledge, derived from basic and medical research, into application for preventive medicine. In order to provide conclusive evidence of the value of preventive procedures, large-scale and costly studies in a realistic community setting are often required. Fortunately a number of these are currently in progress: the Hypertension Detection and Folow-Up Program; The Multiple Risk Factor Intervention Trials; The Diabetic Retinopathy Study; The Aspirin Myocardioinfarction Study; The NCI/ACS

58

Breast Cancer Screening Demonstration Project; and the NCI Community Cancer Control Program. The goals and objectives of these projects are outlined below.

The Hypertension Detection and Follow-Up Program (HDFP)

The specific aims of this research program funded by NHLI are:

1. To assess the ability of a program of Stepped Care vs. Regular Care with long-term antihypertensive therapy and appropriate medical management to reduce mortality and morbidity associated with elevated blood pressure in the general population. In the Stepped Care approach medications are prescribed in a stepwise manner beginning with the least toxic drugs and adding more potent (and potentially more toxic) medications as necessary to achieve goal diastolic blood pressure without intolerable side effects and always with the least number of medicines possible.

2. To assess the effects of this Stepped Care program vs. Regular Care on key intermediate measurements related to risk of major cardiovascular complications in hypertensive patients.

3. To monitor and evaluate the toxic and side effects of antihypertensive medication in the Stepped Care group.

4. With total mortality as the primary end point to assess our ability through Stepped Care to influence life expectancy in the populations screened.

The program is expected, more generally, to enhance knowledge regarding specific means and requirements for accomplishing effective therapy of hypertension in a fashion widely applicable to the community at large. With early deaths from hypertension one of the largest single preventable types of death in this country, the importance of this trial is obvious in establishing what can be done with a large ambulant population on whom very little selection has been exercised except for the presence of hypertension.

Multi-Risk Factor Intervention Trial

The Multi-Risk Factor Intervention Trial (MRFIT) is a cooperative study involving a total of 20 clinical centers with funding from the National Heart and Lung Institute. Patient recruitment is presently under way and expected to be completed by the spring of 1975 with an overall recruitment goal of between 11,000 and 12,000. Each individual clinic is expected to recruit a total of 600 patients. The objectives of MRFIT are as follows:

1. The primary objective of the Multiple Risk Factor Intervention Trial is to determine whether, for a group of men at high risk of death

from coronary heart disease, a special intervention program will result in a significant reduction in mortality from coronary heart disease. To achieve this objective, a screening program will be conducted to identify approximately 12,000 men aged 35–64 who

    a. are in the upper 10 percent of risk of death from coronary heart disease based on risk factors of elevated serum cholesterol, elevated diastolic blood pressure, and cigarette smoking,

    b. do not have preexisting, definite clinical coronary heart disease, or other specified causes for exclusion, and

    c. are willing to commit themselves to a six-year intervention program.

2. A second objective is to determine the effect of the special intervention program on other major end points, in particular, the effect on coronary heart disease incidence (nonfatal myocardial infarction and sudden coronary heart disease mortality), cardiovascular mortality, and total mortality (deaths from all causes).

3. Additional objectives are:

    a. to evaluate to the extent the data allow the effect of this intervention on specific subgroups of the randomized population.

    b. To determine incidence and type of any undesirable or toxic effects of the special intervention program.

    c. To enhance knowledge concerning effective and efficient methods for controlling major risk factors in free-living, apparently healthy, coronary-prone, middle-aged American men and for changing the living and health habits of such men and their immediate families.

    d. To enhance knowledge concerning effective and efficient methods for determining risk, evaluating end points, elucidating the course of prognosis of coronary heart disease, and analyzing data for preventive trials in the free-living population.

The Diabetic Retinopathy Study

The Diabetic Retinopathy Study (DRS) is a contract-supported project from the National Eye Institute. The DRS is a cooperative study involving a total of 15 clinical centers designed to evaluate whether or not photocoagulation therapy is a useful means of preserving vision in patients with diabetic retinopathy. Only diabetics with visual acuity of 20/100 or better in each eye, but with evidence of proliferative retinopathy in both eyes, are eligible for enrollment. Patients enrolled are randomly assigned to treatment with either the argon laser or xenon arc. Only one eye is treated with the modality indicated by the random assignment while the other eye remains untreated and serves as a control for evaluation. Patient follow-up is scheduled through 1979 on the anticipated 1,600 study projects.

Aspirin Myocardial Infarction Study

The Aspirin Myocardial Infarction Study (AMIS) is a National Heart and Lung Institute contract-supported clinical trial. The purpose of this trial is to determine whether regular use of aspirin will significantly reduce mortality and other parameters in men and women who have had at least one electrocardiographically documented myocardial infarction.

A total of 30 clinical centers are scheduled to begin the enrollment of approximately 3,500 participants in June, 1975, with recruitment expected to last one year. Each patient will then be followed under a standard protocol for a minimum of three years, unless the study data indicate convincing evidence of beneficial or adverse treatment effects prior to that time. Major end points to be observed include overall mortality, death due to coronary heart disease or stroke, and the occurrence of nonfatal myocardial infarction or stroke.

Breast Cancer Detection Demonstration Projects

A cooperative program, cosponsored by the American Cancer Society and the National Cancer Institute, is designed to demonstrate on a large scale to the medical profession and to the public how valuable mammography, thermography, and clinical examination are in screening for breast cancer. Funds for this program are provided by grants from the ACS, and by contracts with the NCI. The program will extend for at least two years of screening plus five years of follow-up, with at least 5,000 asymptomatic women being screened annually at each of 27 institutions. The screenees will be recruited from the population at large with an emphasis on lower socioeconomic strata, utilizing the volunteer corps of the ACS to the maximum extent. The objectives are as follows:

1. To find out if research methods for the detection of breast cancer can be applied to the general population through regular medical channels.

2. To determine if a negative thermogram is sufficient to preclude the use of clinical examination and mammography in the detection of breast cancer.

3. To determine if American Cancer Society volunteers can provide a population of women for screening with adequate follow-up phases of this study.

4. To determine or confirm the observation that nonpalpable breast

cancer, promptly treated, will provide more years free of known disease than waiting for palpable evidence of disease.

5. To evaluate the effect of ACS literature on the teaching of breast self-examination in an effort to find out if women continue self-examination of the breast and if they do not, then why?

6. To try to define again high risk groups for breast cancer.

Success in these projects will be measured by:

1. Number of nonpalpable breast cancers detected.

2. Prolonged life (i.e., five years survival without evidence of disease) of patients with nonpalpable breast cancer, compared with patients who have palpable breast cancer.

3. Number of women screened in these projects who continue self-examination of the breast, as compared with experience in other studies.

4. Mortality rates of women with nonpalpable breast cancer as compared to women with palpable tumors.

Cancer Control and Rehabilitation Program

The Division of Cancer Control and Rehabilitation of the National Cancer Institute is developing an extensive program of applied research to identify new methods, knowledge, and techniques of cancer control; to field test and evaluate their potential usefulness; and if found valuable to demonstrate the applicability of control techniques in large-scale community environments, and then promote their widespread utilization throughout the country. Communities are being selected which have the capacity to institute changes that might influence cancer morbidity and mortality on a large scale. Such trials are essential if cancer prevention is to move from assumptions to scientifically tested results and then to general community application.

V. Conclusions and Recommendations

While the early history of preventive medicine was mainly concerned with eradication of specific communicable diseases, modern preventive medicine focuses on conditions that are precursors to the current major fatal diseases. These conditions include certain anatomic, physiological, chemical, immunologic, and bacterial aspects of the human organism, such as carcinoma-in-situ, high blood pressure, high blood cholesterol, susceptibility to measles, and infection with gonorrhea. The conditions of importance to preventive medicine also include certain habits such as cigarette smoking and excessive use of alcohol that have been identified as precursors of disease.

Enough is known about these physical and behavioral risk factors and their control to justify a major effort to incorporate an attack on them as an integral part of personal health services. This new thrust toward health maintenance, based upon finding and controlling the conditions that lead to disease, constitutes modern preventive medicine.

This approach to health maintenance should take the form of a minimum set of physical and counseling procedures designed specifically for various age and sex groups. Rather than a "general, annual checkup" it is now possible to outline the precise minimum steps that should be taken at certain critical periods of human development, i.e., at pregnancy, infancy, school entry, puberty, entry into adult life, and every five years during early and middle adult years, and every two years thereafter. These minimum sets of preventive medical services should be made available to all persons as the basic approach to health maintenance. Special additional procedures should be included for individuals known to be at higher risk for particular conditions, e.g., conditions associated with certain genetic background or environmental exposures.

At any one time the precise items to be incorporated into the sets of preventive medical services must be determined upon the basis of (1) scientific evidence concerning the significance of the conditions and the effectiveness of detecting and controlling them, and (2) prudent interpretation of the evidence, especially in respect to the appropriateness of wide-scale application. Ideally, procedures and measures should be adopted only when the scientific basis for their use is clear-cut; every effort should be made to extend and refine understanding to that end. Upon occasion, however, as in the whole of medicine, judgments will vary concerning the significance of available knowledge. At such times prudence, based on concurrence of expert opinion, should prevail.

The fact that four separate bodies of American experts in preventive medicine have concurred so completely on the concept and even the details presented in this report indicates that a system for aiming at such prudent judgment is available.

Obviously, as scientific evidence accumulates adjustments should be made in the sets of preventive medical services. It is intended to be a dynamic process of refining and extending preventive medical services.

Applications of the sets of preventive medical services outlined will, of course, be effective only to the extent that conditions found to need attention are vigorously pursued. For that reason the services, while they may be performed by a variety of agencies, should be linked into a comprehensive system of personal health services. The latter, hopefully aimed in the future primarily at health maintenance, also must include all necessary medical diagnosis and therapy. Probably the most effective way to accomplish this is to organize comprehensive personal health services for well-defined segments of the population, thus creating a way of getting the services to all individuals for whom the personal health services system has assumed responsibilty.

Financial arrangements for the preventive medical services should assure equal and uniform access for all members of the population, without any hindrance to access created by a payment mechanism. That means no "deductibles" or "coinsurance" payment imposed at the time the preventive medical services are obtained, since such payments have been shown to inhibit access.

Research and development aimed at expanding and refining the scientific base for preventive medicine should be intensified throughout the scientific community. Only in this way can the full potential be realized. In particular large-scale demonstrations of measures that show promise should be undertaken, in order to assess effectiveness and cost factors. Because of the crucial importance of epidemiology to preventive medicine and the severe lack of personnel skilled in that field, training of epidemiologists should be promptly expanded.

References

Selected References on Hypertension Screening

[1] Veterans Administration Cooperative Study Group on Antihypertensive Agents, "Effects of Treatment on Morbidity in Hypertension: Results in Patients with Diastolic Blood Pressures Averaging 115 through 129 mm Hg," *JAMA* 202:1028–1034, 1967.

Results of a randomized double-blind study of antihypertensive drugs vs. placebos in 143 patients with clinic diastolic blood pressures of 115 through 129 mm Hg demonstrates the value of antihypertensive drug therapy (thiazides, reserpine, and hydralazine) in preventing morbidity and mortality. The patients were admitted into the study from April 1964 to December 1966 and observations ended in May 1967—38 percent of the patients were observed for two years or more. During this period 27 morbid events (four deaths) developed in the placebo group as compared to two (no deaths) in the actively treated patients.

[2] Veterans Administration Cooperative Study Group on Antihypertensive Agents, "Effects of Treatment on Morbidity in Hypertension II. Results in Patients with Diastolic Blood Pressure Averaging 90 through 114 mm Hg," *JAMA* 213:1143–1152, 1970.

The report presents the results of a prospective, controlled trial of drug treatment on morbidity and mortality in a group of 380 patients with a median age of 49 years (from a selected population) with mild or moderate hypertension whose initial diastolic blood pressure averaged 90 through 114 mm Hg. The patients were followed for up to 5.5 years, average 3.3 years, and during this period 56 morbid events (19 deaths related to hypertensive or atherosclorotic complications) developed in the control group as compared to 22 (eight deaths) in the treated patients. The difference in the incidence of morbid events between control and treated patients was less clear-cut in the patients with diastolic blood pressure below 105 mm Hg (21 vs. 14).

[3] Veterans Administration Cooperative Study Group on Antihypertensive Agents, "Effects of Treatment on Morbidity in Hypertension III. Influence of Age, Diastolic Pressure, and Prior Cardiovascular Disease: Further Analysis of Side Effects," *Circulation* 45:991–1004, 1972.

Additional data are presented from the VA study, for male patients with diastolic blood pressures averaging 90–114 mm Hg. Age and presence of cardiovascular-renal abnormalities at entry appeared to strongly influence subsequent attack rates, whereas entry level of blood pressure had a realtively smaller effect on attack rates. On the other hand, effectiveness of treatment appeared to be most influenced by the initial level of blood pressure. Patients with prerandomized diastolic blood pressure in the range of 90 to 104 mm Hg derived relatively little benefit from treatment unless they had cardiovascular-renal abnormalities at entry or were over 50 years of age.

[4] Hypertension Study Group, "Guidelines for the Detection, Diagnosis, and Management of Hypertensive Populations," *Circulation* 44:A-263–A-272, 1971.

Community control of hypertension represents a challenge to American medicine; the scope of the problem is reflected by the lack of adequate diagnostic and therapeutic facilities to manage the case load and the relatively high prevalence of hypertension in economically underprivileged areas including overcrowded urban centers. However, in the long run it should be less expensive to control hypertension than to care for those who become disabled and economically unproductive as a consequence of the disease. In most instances community hypertension control activities will be, and ideally should be, part of a comprehensive health maintenance service. The traditional, detailed and costly diagnostic evaluation of the hypertensive is neither pertinent nor desirable. Rather it is feasible and medically sound to use an effective and relatively inexpensive battery of diagnostic tests that will rule out most cases of secondary hypertension and provide sufficient information to initiate and guide safe and effective medical management.

[5] H.A. Kahn, J.H. Medalie, H.N. Neufeld, E. Riss, and U. Goldbourt, "The Incidence of Hypertension and Associated Factors: The Israel Ischemic Heart Disease Study," *Am. Heart J.* 84:171–182, 1972.

In a study of male Israeli civil service workers, five-year incidence rates of hypertension (using the WHO definition) were found to increase with age and varied from a low of 28 per 1,000 for those born in Africa to a high of 76 per 1,000 for those born in Southern Europe. Data are presented in support of a hypothesis that the size of the family group living together is inversely related to the risk of developing hypertension. Other factors found associated with hypertension incidence (all positively) were weight/height ratio, skinfolds, serum uric acid, pulse rate, cigarette smoking, and prolongation and suppression of feelings following conflicts in certain life situations.

[6] J.D. Abernathy, "The Australian National Blood Pressure Study," *Med. J. Aust.* 1:821–824, 1974.

A description of the plan of the Australian National Blood Pressure Study is presented. The screening program commenced in June 1973 and the primary question to be addressed is whether pharmacological treatment of people with mild hypertension (diastolic blood pressure 95–109 mm Hg) improves prognosis. It is stated that the U.S. Veterans Study referred to a more severe degree of hypertension than equivalent blood pressure levels determined at casual examination since a considerable proportion of the VA subjects had preexisting cardiovascular or renal complications.

[7] A. Apostolides, J.R. Hebel, M.S. McDill, and M.M. Henderson, "High Blood Pressure: Its Care and Consequences in Urban Centers," *Int. J. Epidemiol.* 3:105–117, 1974.

The results of a special secondary prevention program for hypertension were compared to those of usual medical care available to patients with high blood pressure. The extent of the problem in disadvantaged communities, the diminishing return for added control activities, the relatively greater impact of special care at high diastolic blood pressure levels, and the overwhelming contribution of behavioral modification to program success, lead the authors to question the basic decision to extend the application of the available secondary prevention tool to control this major disorder.

[8] D. Short, (Letter), "Diagnosis and Treatment of Hypertension," *Lancet* 2:645, 1974.

The VA study did not in fact demonstrate that treatment was of value in mild hypertension; indeed it did not really deal with mild hypertension at all. Although the patients had diastolic pressures within the range 90–114, these pressures were recorded under basal or mean basal conditions, and at the fifth phase. This latter point is not clear from the published reports, but it has been confirmed by the Chairman of the VA group. Thus, the range 90–114 in the VA study corresponds to at least 100–124 in clinical practice.

[9] K.L. Stuart, P. Desai, and A. Lalsingh, "Approach to Assessment of Risk Factors in Mild Hypertension," *Br. Med. J.* 2:195–198, 1974.

The recognition and attempted treatment of all subjects with mild hypertension would pose problems of both practicability and ethical justification. Thus two major questions would have to be answered before routine treatment of this group of people could be instituted. The first relates to the recognition of subjects with mild hypertension who may be at greatest risk, and the second is whether these high-risk subjects once identified could be shown to benefit from lowering of the blood pressure. In this preliminary study some of the factors that may be of value in identifying high-risk subjects were investigated: enlarged heart, high serum cholesterol levels, effort pain, ECG abnormalities, and high systolic blood pressure. Any two or more of these possible risk factors were found to occur significantly more often in an index group consisting of 22 patients with fatal or morbid end points (95–114 mm Hg initial diastolic pressure) than in a control group of 22 subjects chosen at random with the same diastolic pressure, age and sex distribution (both followed for five years). High systolic pressure was the only significant factor when each was assessed separately.

[10] E.A. Lew, "High Blood Pressure, Other Risk Factors and Longevity: The Insurance Viewpoint," *Am. J. Med.* 55:281–294, 1973.

Follow-up studies among insured persons carried out over a period of nearly 50 years have established that untreated blood pressures in excess of 140/90 mm Hg are associated with a significant degree of extra mortality in the long run; for instance, in men under 40 with casual pressures of 150/100 mortality was approximately 325 percent that of standard insured risks, whereas corresponding men aged 40 and over showed a mortality of about 225 percent. Such excess mortality increases with rise in blood pressure and is greater in the presence of other impairments or complications.

[11] E.D. Freis, "Age, Race, Sex and Other Indices of Risk in Hypertension," *Am. J. Med.* 55:275–280, 1973.

Among the various criteria used in evaluating the prognosis of hypertensive patients the level of the diastolic blood pressure averaged over three or more visits is the important index. Other indices also are useful and are essential in deciding on treating patients with average diastolic blood pressures below 105 mm Hg. Male sex, young age, and black race are all associated with increased risk of morbidity and mortality. The lability of the hypertension is another indicator of risk. Patients with labile hypertension—high casual in relation to basal blood pressure—have a better prognosis than those who do not.

[12] R.B. Singer, "To Treat or Not to Treat," *J. Chron. Dis.* 28:125–134, 1975.

It is predicted that 1.8 million excess deaths occur over a 10-year period in hypertensives aged 35–64 when hypertensive mortality rates are compared with normotensive ones. Three-quarters of the excess deaths would be anticipated among definite hypertensives (over 160 systolic or 95 diastolic) and the remaining one-quarter among borderline hypertensives (under 160/95 and over 140/90). These two groups are almost equal in size, however, with more than 11 million people each.

[13] S.H. Zinner, L.F. Martin, F. Sacks, B. Rosner, and E.H. Kass, "A Longitudinal Study of Blood Pressure in Childhood," *Am. J. Epid.* 100:437–442, 1975.

This study (609 children aged 6–18) found that 65 percent of those children with initial scores greater than one standard deviation unit above the mean had positive blood pressure scores when reexamined at follow-up four years later, and that similar stratification persists in those with lower blood pressures. This is consistent with observations made in much older adults and suggests that stratification of blood pressures in relation to peer groups begins in childhood.

[14] J. Stamler and F.H. Epstein, "Coronary Heart Disease: Risk Factors as Guides to Preventive Action," *Prev. Med.* 1:27–48, 1972.

Hypercholesterolemia, hypertension, and cigarette smoking are major risk factors for coronary heart disease. Their preeminence as predictors is confirmed by multivariate analysis, using a series of additional factors and testing their relative importance by a modified form of discriminant analysis. The overwhelming weight of evidence implicating these risk factors makes it mandatory for physicians in practice as well as those in public health to incorporate detection in regular examinations of adults, including the asymptomatic.

[15] D.L. Sackett, "Screening for Disease: Cardiovascular Diseases," *Lancet* 2:1189–1191, 1974.

Based on a review of criteria which must be satisfied before launching mass screening programs, it is concluded the community-wide screening is not rational at the present time. Although we can identify individuals at risk, methods of treatment and compliance with these therapeutic measures are still so unsatisfactory that there is little point in identification by screening.

[16] S.B. Stokes, G.H. Payne, and T. Cooper, "Hypertension Control—The Challenge of Patient Education," *N. Engl. J. Med.* 289:1369–1370, 1973.

There are over 23 million Americans with hypertension (blood pressure over 160/95 mm Hg). On the basis of a survey only 61 percent of the 99 percent who have ever had their blood pressure checked were told anything about their blood pressure; 50 percent of the hypertensive population are unaware of their condition.

[17] J. Fry, "Natural History of Hypertension—A Case For Selective Non-Treatment," *Lancet* 2:431–433, 1974.

Based on 20 years experience in a general practice it is concluded that there is no strong case for hypertensives first diagnosed over age 60 to be treated with specific hypotensives.

[18] Special Task Force on Hypertension, Regional Medical Program Service, *Medical Basis for Comprehensive Community Hypertension Control Program*, DHEW, July 1973.

[19] American Heart Association, Subcommittee on Reduction of Risk of Heart Attack and Stroke, *Stroke Risk Handbook—Estimating Risk of Stroke in Daily Practice*, New York, American Heart Association, 1974.

Selected References on Screening for Cervical Cancer by Cytology

[1] J.E. MacGregor and S. Teper (Letter), "Screening for Cervical Cancer," *Lancet* 1:1221, 1974.

Screening in the northeast region of Scotland started in 1960. About 90 percent of the female population of Aberdeen City over 20 years of age have been screened at least once. There has been a significant fall in the incidence of squamous cervical cancer in Aberdeen (32.0 per 100,000 in 1961 and 16.2 per 100,000 in 1971). Between 1961 and 1971 the death-rates from cervical cancer for women aged 20 years and over fell from 24.0 per 100,000 to 17.2 per 100,000 (and from 18.4 to 10.1 for women aged 20–54). This fall has occurred sooner than might be expected. Through screening carcinoma in situ is detected 10–15 years before it would be present clinically; however several cases have been detected at the symptomless but microinvasive stage and without diagnosis and treatment these women would have died in their late 60s.

[2] S. Timonen, U. Nieminen, and T. Kauraniemi (Letter), "Cervical Screening," *Lancet* 1:401–402, 1974.

A cervical screening program was started in Finland at the beginning of the 1960s. Every woman receives a personal invitation to screening at five-year intervals, generally, from the age of 30 or 35. Attendance in the whole country has been 78 percent. A decline in the incidence of cervical carcinoma has been noticeable since 1967 (14.5 per 100,000 in 1970). Before introduction of mass screening the incidence of cervical carcinoma proved to be remarkably stable (16–18 per 100,000) or perhaps slightly rising.

[3] L. Breslow, "Early Case-Finding, Treatment, and Mortality from Cervix and Breast Cancer," *Prev. Med.* 1:141–152, 1972.

The accelerating decline in cervix cancer mortality in California during the 1960s appears to have been due to the widespread use of the cytologic test beginning in the late 1950s, resulting in discovery of the disease during the early stages when cure is more likely. Based on evidence that the in situ stage may persist on the average as long as 10 years and that about 90 percent of deaths from cervix cancer (invasive stage) occur within five years of diagnosis, it seems reasonable to expect an impact on cervix cancer mortality only about 5–10 years after cytology is first widely applied, and this has evidently occurred in California.

[4]D.A. Boyes, J. Knowlelden, and A.J. Phillips, "The Evaluation of Cancer Control Measures," *Br. J. Cancer* 28:105–107, 1973.

A brief report of the conclusion reached in a UICC symposium held in September 1972 to evaluate the effectiveness of mass screening programs. A consensus view was reached on the value of screening for lesions of the cervix, breast, and stomach. It was agreed that screening tests for other sites were not yet ready for application, either because the results were not clear-cut or because no effective treatment was available for the condition detected.

[5]L.J. Kinlen and R. Doll, "Trends in Mortality from Cancer of the Uterus in Canada and in England and Wales," *Brit. J. Prev. Soc. Med.* 27:146–149, 1973.

Comparable data from 1966–1971 were examined with previous data from 1955–65 to determine if the extensive cervical cancer screening program in British Columbia has been followed by any appreciable change in the mortality from cervix cancer. (In 1962 the number of smears taken per 100 women was 23 in British Columbia and four in the rest of Canada; in 1967 the rates were 41 and 19 respectively. Data are not available on the number of women who have been screened). The results show that the mortality from cervix cancer has declined materially in the last 10 years, particularly under 45 years of age, but that there is very little difference between the experience in British Columbia, Ontario, and other parts of Canada. Only at ages 45–64 does British Columbia appear to have had any appreciable advantage. However, it does not necessarily follow that even this difference can be attributed to the screening program.

[6]G.H. Green and J.W. Donovan, "The Natural History of Cervical Carcinoma in situ," *J. Obstet. Gynec. Brit. Cwlth.* 77:1–9, 1970.

Of a total of 576 patients with cervical carcinoma in situ, 75 have shown evidence of persistent disease after various initial treatments. None of the 75 have developed invasive cervical cancer during follow-up. The 75 patients were representative of the total series of 576 with respect to age and parity. Their mean follow-up time was 53 months (range 13 to 141 months). This result is used to obtain confidence limits for the probability with which carcinoma in situ becomes invasive and for the period after which it does so.

[7]K.J. Randall, "Cancer Screening by Cytology," *Lancet* 4:1303–1304, 1974.

A brief review of screening which concludes that cervical cytology offered as a selective screening procedure can significantly reduce the mortality from carcinoma of the cervix. Recognition is given to the fact that those most at risk are the least likely to attend regularly, or at all, for testing.

[8]J. Wakefield, R. Yule, A. Smith and A.M. Adelstein, "Relation of Abnormal Cytological Smears and Carcinoma of Cervix Uteri to Husband's Occupation," *Br. Med. J.* 2:142–143, 1973.

An analysis of the cytological records of almost 300,000 women shows that the rates of postive/suspicious findings from population screening are highly correlated with the rates of mortality from cancer of the cervix among women in the years before screening began when both are distributed according to the occupation of the husband. The correlation holds for various occupational groupings and for all the individual units in which there are more than 1,000 women. The findings described here highlight the specificity of these rates (both clinical and preclinical) in groupings narrower than social class. This evidence strengthens the case for believing that the histological changes noted in screening are related to the cancer and that the most likely explanation is that the cytological changes, and in particular carcinoma in situ, are precursors of clinical cancer.

[9] L.W. Coppleson and B. Brown, "Estimation of the Screening Error Rates from the Observed Detection Rates in Repeated Cervical Cytology," *Am. J. Obstet. Gynecol.* 119:953–958, 1974.

Third and fourth observed apparent incidence rates were successively smaller that the initial observed incidence rate (the second screening rate) in some studies where repeated screening was used to detect dysplasia, carcinoma in situ, and invasive cancer. Since the false-negative error rate in cervical screening is known to be high, it was suspected that this error, as it was expressed in successive screenings, was causing the step-down effect. A model was designed to test this hypothesis and error rates were calculated by least-squares fit of the model to the observed data. False-negative error rates of 40 percent for dysplasia, 20–45 percent for carcinoma in situ and 24 percent for invasive cancer were found.

[10] E. Wachtel, "Screening for Cervical Cancer," *Practitioner* 211:137–142, 1973.

A review of the literature leaves the author with the opinion that the beneficial effects of mass screening are clearly shown. Attention is given to the reliability of a cytological report, the relationship between carcinoma-in-situ and invasive cancer, level of participation in screening programs, and the results of population screening of the incidence of invasive cancer of the cervix and on mortality.

[11] C.E. Lewis, "Consumer Control of Carcinoma of the Cervix," *Am. J. Obstet. Gynecol.* 119:669–674, 1974.

A study was carried out to determine the extent of compliance of women with recommendation of physicians for annual Papanicolaou examinations. Eighty-six of 22,464 clinic patients seen at a teaching hospital returned for five successive annual examinations. The average annual rate of return was approximately 25 percent. Review of office records from a group pracitice of specialists providing care for upper-middle class women demonstrated that 48 percent returned for an annual smear when letters were written to remind patients that they were due for such an examination.

[12] E.G. Knox, "A Simulation For Screening Procedures," in G. McLachlan (ed); *Problems and Progress in Medical Care*, 9th Series, London, Oxford University Press, 1973, pp. 17–55.

A simulation model is developed in relation to the evaluation of options related to cervical cytology screening programmes. The simulation model is used to test the effect on lives saved of variations in the natural history of disease, the age at which screening is initiated, the number of tests offered and the acceptability of the test in terms of percentage participating in the program. Based on the simulation exercise the following conclusions were reached: (a) ignorance of the exact natural history of disease, which is of some importance when small resources are deployed for screening, becomes crucially important as investment rises; (b) the best deployment of a screening program is around age 40 and the marginal costs required to effect any increase in death saved mount rapidly between five and 10 test offers and the discrepancies between estimates based on (two) different models of natural disease history are particularly wide at this point; and (c) the difficulties of achieving high levels of control have probably been underestimated in the past—sooner or later a point will be reached where the resources are better spent elsewhere.

[13] J.B. Thorn, J.E. MacGregor, E.M. Russell, and K. Swanson, "Costs of Detecting and Treating Cancer of the Uterine Cervix in North-East Scotland in 1971," *Lancet* 1:674–676, 1975.

Based on the experience of the Aberdeen cytology service, the cost of detecting and treating a case of cancer of the uterine cervix at a preclinical stage is slightly less than for inpatient treatment of a clinical case. If mass screening were abandoned, cytology would almost certainly continue for women referred to the hospital with symptoms, and if the cost of taking and examining these smears is taken into account, the cost per clinical case nearly doubles.

[14] *Cancer Facts and Figures*, New York, American Cancer Society, 1975.

[15] L. Dickinson, M.E. Massey, E.H. Soules, and L.T. Kurland, "Evaluation of the Effectiveness of Cytologic Screening for Cervical Cancer," *Mayo Clinic Proc.* 47:534–544, 1972.

[16] S. Timonen, U. Nieminen, and T. Kauraniemi, "Mass Screening for Cervical Carcinoma in Finland," *Annales Chirurgiae et Gynaecologiae Fenniae* 63:104–112, 1974.

[17] M. Gronroos, J. Tyrkko, O. Tarvi, and L. Rauramo, "Experience of a Continuing Mass Screening Programme," *Annales Chirurgiae et Gynaecologiae Fenniae* 63:470–478, 1974.

[18] K. Grunfeld, O. Horwitz, and B. Lysgaard-Hansen, "Evaluation of Mortality Data for Cervical Cancer With Special Reference to Mass Screening Programs, Denmark, 1961–1971," *Am. J. Epid.* 101:265–275, 1975.

Selected References on Screening for Breast Cancer

[1] S. Shapiro, P. Strax, L. Venet, and W. Venet, "Changes in 5-year Breast Cancer Mortality in a Breast Cancer Screening Program," in *Seventh National Cancer Conference Proceedings,* Philadelphia, J.B. Lippincott Co., 1972, pp. 663–678.

This paper provides data, covering a follow-up period of five years, which indicate that women in an annual breast cancer screening program with mammography and clinical examination have a one-third lower mortality from breast cancer than a similarly constituted control group. Reduction in mortality is concentrated entirely among women over 50 years of age. Five-year death rates for all other causes of mortality are almost identical for study and control groups. Detection by mammography was especially important in contributing to this reduction in mortality due to breast cancer. A critical element of the investigation is that the study group included all women who were offered screening (31,000) whether or not they accepted (65 percent appeared for initial screening exams).

[2] S. Shapiro, J.D. Goldberg, and G.B. Hutchinson, "Lead Time in Breast Cancer Detection and Implications for Periodicity of Screening," *Am. J. Epidemiol.* 100:357–366, 1974.

The experience in the HIP breast cancer screening study was used to estimate the average lead time gained through screening in the detection of breast cancer among women aged 40–64 years. The statistical models that were applied suggest that the average lead time is about a year; at the initial examination, the gain is estimated at seven months; at subsequent screenings conducted about a year apart, the gain is estimated at 11–13 months. The HIP screening project reduction of five-year mortality from breast cancer occurred among women aged 50 and over and not among those under 50. A matter of considerable importance now being investigated is whether the lead time estimates differ for these two groups.

[3] S. Shapiro, "Screening for Early Detection of Cancer and Heart Disease," *Bull. N.Y. Acad. Med.* 51:80–95, 1975.

Primarily a review of screening for breast cancer based on the HIP study. It is concluded that although it is unrealistic at this time to expect a rapid spread of screening programs for breast cancer to cover major segments of the female population, two types of activities should be carried out simultaneously over the next few years: (1) expansion of the availability of screening for breast cancer, either in conjunction with multiphasic examinations or in single-purpose examinations, and (2) further research to improve the efficiency of screening programs, to decrease costs, and to conserve physicians' time.

[4] E.G. Knox, "Simulation Studies of Breast Cancer Screening Programmes" (Manuscript prepared for publication) 1975.

This study is an exploration, using computer simulation, of various conditions of interest in a breast screening service and indicates the following: i) A straightforward extension of the HIP pattern of screening will encounter diminishing returns and a fall in the marginal value of additional tests; ii) The marginal value of added mammography over palpation alone will fall as the service is extended and will reach a point where additional mammographies may be doing more harm than good; iii) Pre-selection techniques, even when not very selective, can greatly increase the economy of a screening scheme despite a possible tendency to select women with less tractable tumours; iv) The value of pre-selection techniques tends to increase as the service extends; they are not to be seen simply as a stop-gap during an initial period of limited resources; v) Having regard to the limited acceptability of screening procedures, their high costs, the pattern of diminishing returns and the hazards of radiation and of unnecessary biopsy, a reasonable service target (within present technology) may be a reduction of breast cancer mortality by about one-tenth.

[5] A.H. Dowdy, W.F. Barker, L.D. Lagasse, L. Sperling, L.J. Zeldis, and W.P. Longmire, Jr., "Mammography as a Screening Method for the Examination of Large Populations," *Cancer* 28:1558–1562, 1971.

Three years of experience in a UCLA screening program for breast cancer in women 40 years of age and over are reviewed. The authors note that due to the lack of adequately trained professional and allied health personnel, a massive screening program on a national scale is unwarranted and would be unproductive at this time.

[6] I.G. Furnival, H.J. Stewart, J.M. Weddell, P. Dovey, I.H. Gravelle, K.T. Evans, and A.P.M. Forrest, "Accuracy of Screening Methods for the Diagnosis of Breast Cancer," *Br. Med. J.* 4:461–463, 1970.

Clinical examination, thermography, and 70-mm mammography were performed in 891 patients—414 presented to hospital with symptoms of breast disease and 477 were asymptomatic. Comparison of these methods showed that the diagnostic accuracy of thermography and 70-mm mammography does not approach that of clinical examination in patients with symptomatic disease. It is concluded that neither thermography nor 70-mm mammography is suitable for use alone in the diagnosis of breast disease, nor can either method be used in isolation as a screening procedure.

[7] B. Friedman, P. Barker, and L. Lipworth, "The Influence of Medicaid and Private Health Insurance on the Early Diagnosis of Breast Cancer," *Medical Care* 11:485–490, 1973.

Several medical, social, and economic variables have an influence on the stage of cancer at the time it is first treated. This paper investigates the independent effects of insurance coverage. Based on data for breast cancers first treated in 1970 occurring to women in a large Massachusetts population and first treated in 1970, the results do not support the view that eliminating the direct expense to consumers of medical care is a meaningful stimulus to the early diagnosis of serious illness.

[8] R.L.A. Kirch, and M. Klein, "Examination Schedules for Breast Cancer," *Cancer* 33:1444–1450, 1974.

Annual breast cancer examination programs are known to yield favorable survival statistics, presumably because of early disease detection, and earlier detection may be possible if examinations are scheduled more frequently. Using a mathematical model, calculations indicate that a semiannual examination program may detect cancer three months earlier than an annual examination program, and there appears to be only a slight economic advantage (2-3 percent) if examination frequency is a function of age rather than fixed according to a periodic schedule.

[9] D. Kodlin, "A Note on the Cost-Benefit Problem in Screening for Breast Cancer," *Meth. Inform. Med.* 11:242-247, 1972.

Using a series of biometrical arguments and very crude cost estimates, the author determines that survival results would justify the increased results that might result from mass screening. The analysis is based on single rather than periodic screening and only two disease states—early and progressed—are considered.

[10] A.M. Stark and S. Way, "The Screening of Well Women for the Early Detection of Breast Cancer Using Clinical Examination with Thermography and Mammography," *Cancer* 33:1671-1679, 1974.

A group of 2,684 women, selected as being at higher than average risk of breast cancer, has been screened by clinical examination, thermography, and mammography. The pickup rate for preclinical breast cancer is 19.3 per 1,000.

[11] L.M. Irwig, "Screening for Disease: Breast Cancer," *Lancet* 2:1307, 1974.

A position on screening for breast cancer is summarized. Available methods look promising but technical improvements are needed to reduce cost.

[12] *Cancer Facts and Figures,* New York, American Cancer Society, 1975.

Selected References on Multiphasic Screening

[1] L. Breslow, "An Historical Review of Multiphasic Screening," *Prev. Med.* 2:177-196, 1973.

An historical and detailed review of the development of multiphasic screening and its potential role in health maintenance.

[2] S. Shapiro, "Automated Multiphasic Health Testing: Efficacy of the Concept," *Hospitals* 45:45-48, 1971.

A review of the various viewpoints on multiphasic health screening and ongoing evaluation studies designed to test the efficacy of multiphasic health testing.

[3] E.G. Knox, "Screening for Disease: Multiphasic Screening," *Lancet* 4:1434-1435, 1974.

A review of the definitions of multiphasic screening, objectives, and evaluations in terms of improved mortality or morbidity rates. A review of reported cost per examination and cost expressed in relation to yields is presented. It is stated that genuine health-care objectives of reducing illness of a multiphasic screening scheme examined for effectiveness. In the meantime the view is taken that multiphasic health screening procedures appear to be of little value in medical practice at the present time, particularly in respect of individuals who are apparently well and who are not in hospital.

[4] M.F. Collen, P.H. Kidd, R. Feldman, and J.L. Cutler, Cost Analysis of Multiphasic Screening Program," *N. Eng. J. Med.*, 280:1043-1045, 1969.

Based on cost analysis automated multiphasic screening provides a battery of tests that would cost four or five times as much by traditional nonautomated methods. However, the unit cost per multiphasic screening ($21.32) is inversely related (almost linearly) to the patient load (2,000 per month) and thus reflects economies of scale. The authors conclude that if a decision is made to provide health examinations to large numbers of people, the most efficient and economical means is by the use of automated multitest laboratories.

[5] S. Ramcharan, J. Cutler, R. Feldman, A.B. Siegelaub, B. Campbell, G.D. Friedman, L.G. Dales, and M.F. Collen, "Multiphasic Check-up Evaluation Study 2. Disability and Chronic Disease After Seven Years of Multiphasic Health Check-ups," *Prev. Med.* 2:207–220, 1973.

A controlled trial has been in progress since April 1964 to evaluate the efficacy of the periodic health examination utilizing automated multiphasic testing. After five to seven years, a favorable impact on the health of the older study males compared to the older control males (born during 1910–1919) was evidenced by: (a) a reduction in self-rated disability and reported time lost from work; (b) a greater proportion working; and (c) a lower self-reported utilization of medical services by the sick.

[6] Loring G. Dales, G.D. Friedman, S. Ramacharan, A.B. Siegelaub, B.A. Campbell, R. Feldman, and M.F. Collen, "Multiphasic Check-up Evaluation Study 3. Outpatient Clinic Utilization, Hospitalization, and Mortality Experience After Seven Years," *Prev. Med.* 2:221–235, 1973.

The Multiphasic Check-up Evaluation Study is a controlled clinical trial (persons aged 35–54 at entry) aimed at testing the efficacy of periodic Multiphasic Health Check-ups in preventing or postponing illness, disability, and death. While there has been little difference in utilization of outpatient physician and laboratory services other than those directly connected with the Multiphasic Health Check-ups, the study group subjects have had more diagnoses made. Among the men ages 45–54 at entry, hospital usage has been slightly lower in the study group, while the opposite has been the case among the women ages 45–54 at entry. The overall mortality rate has been slightly lower in the study group (35.6 vs. 39.2 per 1,000 persons for the seven-year period), while for a group of causes of death defined as being potentially postponable or preventable (certain cancers and hypertension associated diseases), the study group mortality rate has been significantly lower (3.7 vs. 7.4).

[7] M.F. Collen, L.G. Dales, G.D. Friedman, C.D. Flagle, R. Feldman, and A.B. Siegelaub, "Multiphasic Check-up Evaluation Study 4. Preliminary Cost Benefit Analysis for Middle-Aged Men," *Prev. Med.* 2:236–246, 1973.

A preliminary cost benefit analysis for a program of urging middle-aged men to take annual Multiphasic Health Check-ups has suggested a net savings of more than $800 per man over a seven-year period among men urged to take the check-ups as compared to men not so urged. This difference principally reflects the lower disability and mortality rates observed for the men who were urged to receive the check-ups. Similar differences have not been demonstrated for women or younger men.

[8] Sam Shapiro "Evaluation of Two Contrasting Types of Screening Programs," *Prev. Med.* 2:266–277, 1973.

HIP is testing whether through AMHT, and the activities generated by it, the anticipated gaps between poverty and nonpoverty groups in the occurrence of health problems can be lessened (i.e., whether the impact of a multiple array of services, automated multiphasic health testing, and follow-up paramedical and medical services on health status and health care behavior is greater among the poor than the rest of the population). Preliminary analysis indicates that a significant gap exists in the occurrence of health problems.

[9] Harriet Trevelyan, "Study to Evaluate the Effects of Multiphasic Screening within General Practice in Britain: Design and Method," *Prev. Med.* 1, 278–294, 1973.

74

Two group practices in London are evaluating the effects of multiphasic screening on health service usage, and the prevalence of certain symptoms, diseases, and disability in individuals between 40 and 64 years of age.

[10] Robert M. Thorner, D. Djordjevic, C. Vuckmanovic, B. Pesic, B. Culafic, and F. Mark, "A Study to Evaluate the Effectiveness of Multiphasic Screening in Yugoslavia," *Prev. Med.* 2:295–301.

A study in Yugoslavia (13,150 individuals aged 30 to 49) is being conducted to evaluate the effect of multiphasic screening in Yugoslavia on mortality, morbidity, absence from work, and utilization of medical services.

[11] M.F. Collen et al., "Dollar Cost For Positive Test For AMHS," *New Eng. J. Med.* 283:459–463, 1970.

[12] J.L. Cutler, S. Ramcharan, R. Feldman, A.B. Siegelaub, B. Campbell, G.D. Friedman, L.G. Dales, and M.F. Collen, "Multiphasic Check-up Evaluation Study 1. Methods and Population," *Prev. Med.* 2:197–206, 1973.

[13] C.K. Canelo, D.M. Bissel, H. Abrams, and L. Breslow, "A Multiphasic Screening Survey in San Jose," *California Med.* 71:1–5, 1949.

[14] E.R. Weinerman, L. Breslow, N.B. Belloc, A. Waybur, and B.K. Milmore, "Multiphasic Screening of Longshoremen with Organized Medical Follow-up," *Am. J. Pub. Health* 42:1552–1567, 1952.

Selected References on the Organization of Health Services

[1] L. Breslow, "The Organization of Personal Health Services," *Milbank Mem. Fund. Q.* 50:365–386, 1972.

A review of the fundamental issues which support the need for a change in the organization of the delivery of health services. Changes in financing by simply providing more funds is hardly worthwhile and may even add to the inflationary trend. The failure to plan effectively for health care and organize it has resulted in major deficiencies as to cost, quality, and consumer satisfaction. Several things are needed for the evaluation of better health care delivery. High on the list is a national commitment, probably in the form of legislation, to make comprehensive health care equally available to all persons.

[2] U.E. Reinhardt, "Proposed Changes in the Organization of Health Care Delivery: An Overview and Critique," *Milbank Mem. Fund. Q.* 51:169–222, 1973.

In this essay various proposals to reform the health care delivery system are explored against the backdrop of pertinent empirical research available at this time. This exploration leads to the disappointing conclusion that far too many of the proposed reorganization schemes—particularly the much touted idea of a nationwide network of presumably competitive health maintenance organizations—appear to have been proffered more on the basis of intuition or faith than on the basis of convincing empirical evidence. The author concludes that a great deal more empirical information needs to be gathered on the behavior of the participants in the health-care sector and on the technical constraints under which that sector operates before one can confidently develop and follow a coherent blueprint for a reorganization of the American health-care system.

[3] V. Navarro, "National Health Insurance and The Strategy for Change," *Milbank Mem. Fund Q.* 51:223–251, 1973.

This paper sounds a note of caution that regardless of the type of national health insurance program Congress will approve from among the proposals now before it, the reorganization and redistribution of health resources required to secure the availability of care for the greatest possible number may be hindered rather than stimulated. Strategies for change will necessarily be limited in their reorganizational and distributive effects, inasmuch as they leave untouched the locus of economic and political power in the health sector; it is argued that this very locus of power precipitated the much-quoted "medical care crisis." The author believes that the locus of power must shift from the private to the public sector, permitting the levels of federal, state, and local government to formulate a mechanism for national and regional health planning in which public agencies would be the ones primarily responsible for planning, regulating, and controlling the distribution of human and physical resources within the health sector. In the light of this recommendation, the present structure for national and regional planning in the United States is described and appraised.

[4] W. Shonick and M.I. Roemer, "HMO Performance: The Recent Evidence," *Milbank Mem. Fund. Q.* 51:271–317, 1973.

Health maintenance organizations (HMOs) are being promoted as a strategy to modify the U.S. health care delivery system toward more economical patterns, encouraging preventive and ambulatory rather than costly hospital services. Evidence suggests that the "prepaid group practice" model of HMO continues to yield lower hospital use, relatively more ambulatory and preventive service, and lower overall costs than conventional open-market fee-for-service patterns. New data point to reduced disability as well as to more favorable consumer attitudes than exist toward conventionally insured private solo practice. HMOs entail hazards of underservicing and distorted risk-selection, but with appropriate public monitoring they constitute an approach to health planning, stressing local initiative, competition, and incentives to self-regulation.

[5] R. Stockton and B. Stuart, "Control over the Utilization of Medical Services," *Milbank Mem. Fund. Q.* 51:341–394, 1973.

During recent years, the health care industry has been characterized by rapid increases in the volume of services delivered. This escalation is in part unjustified by medical need, and has produced a variety of efforts on the part of payers and providers to restrict overuse. In this article the authors consider the issues and problems involved in the control of medical utilization.
It is concluded that most current forms of utilization control suffer from ambiguity of purpose, organizational inefficiency, and undesirable side effects. The authors offer several proposals to correct these shortcomings, but conclude that the only long-range solution to overutilization lies in a more integrated approach to medical resource allocation and a consequent change in the structure of provider and user incentives.

[6] L. Breslow, "Health Maintenance Services in Health Maintenance Organizations," *Assoc. of Teachers of Prev. Med. Newsletter* 19:1–3, 1972; and "Do HMO's Provide Health Maintenance?" *A Delta Omega Lecture*, San Francisco, Nov. 1973.

Data are provided, some derived from population surveys and some from medical records, which support the view that group practice, prepayment plans in California, like Kaiser, have been providing subscribers a greater amount of health maintenance services than have been provided in other types of plans. It is noted that these data reflect the experience of prototype or "first-generation" health maintenance organizations and that many of the 'second-generation' HMOs in California appear to be concentrating on the economic advantage rather than the health maintenance aspect of HMOs.

[7] M. Henderson, "Preventive Medicine Services," *Assoc. of Teachers of Prev. Med. Newsletter* 20:4–7, 1973.

76

The viewpoint is presented that insufficient evidence exists to demonstrate that HMOs will improve the health of people enrolled in them. Requirements of a rigorous evaluation are listed as a measure against which the adequacy of existing evidence can be assessed. It is stressed that the evaluation must focus on prevention of disease and correction of limitations which are measures of health benefit rather than measures of the level of services provided or program input.

[8] D.L. Rabin, and E. Schach, "Medicaid, Morbidity, and Physician Use," *Medicare Care* 13:68–78, 1975.

A Baltimore SMSA household interview of use of health services permitted comparison of use of physician and preventive services controlled for morbidity by Medicaid recipients and two other income groups. Medicaid recipients were sickest and had higher physician use. Physician visit rates were higher for each morbidity category, particularly for Medicaid healthy, who also used more preventive services in two weeks. Higher use of services by Medicaid recipients is accounted for by higher morbidity and increased need and demand for preventive services. Constraints on the use of physician services now most directly affect use of preventive services by those of low income without Medicaid benefits in the Baltimore SMSA.

[9] P.E. Enterline, J.C. McDonald, A.D. McDonald, and V. Henderson, "Physician's Working Hours and Patients Seen Before and After National Health Insurance: 'Free' Medical Care and Medical Practice," *Medical Care* 13:95–103, 1975.

Surveys were made of a sample of physicians before and after the introduction of a national health insurance plan in Montreal, Canada. Although the number of physicians in active practice seemed unaffected by the plan, their average working day was reduced 1.5 hours. Declines ranged from 0.3 hours for general internists to 2.7 hours for general surgeons. The average daily volume of services by physicians in the area also declined because of a decline in telephone consultations, and home and hospital visits. Office visits increased sharply. Changes in the type of services were clearly related to the fee schedule adopted by the government, with large declines in services for which payment was probably inadequate in relation to physician's time required. If the fee schedule reflected actual collections prior to the health insurance plan, then gross physician income increased as the result of redirecting services to better paying activities.

[10] T.W. Bice, D.L. Rabin, B.H. Starfield, and K.L. White, "Economic Class and Use of Physician Services," *Medical Care* 11:287–296, 1973.

Two assertions about the effects of economic class on use of physician services are tested. It was expected that the net price of services would be more highly related to use among the poor than among high income persons, and that noneconomic predisposing factors would be more highly related to preventive use than to all types of use combined. These assertions were tested using data from a household survey of the Baltimore Standard Metropolitan Statistical Area. Multivariate analyses of two dichotomous dependent variables support both assertions.

[14] E.W. Brian and S.F. Gibbens, "California's Medi-Cal Copayment Experiment, Chapter IV Findings of the Study," *Medical Care* 12 (Supplement): 27–53, 1974.

The results of an attempt to evaluate the impact of a copayment mechanism on utilization and costs under California's Medi-Cal Copayment Experiment. A significant finding in the experiment is that the copay group used preventive services much less frequently than the noncopay group.

[12] M.I. Roemer, C.E. Hopkins, L. Carr, and F. Gartside, "Co-Payments For Ambulatory Care: Penny-Wise and Pound-Foolish," (prepared for publication) 1974.

Reports that copayment reduced use of ambulatory care, but as a result an elevated hospitalization rate was noted in the co-pay group. Short-term savings in lower ambulatory care were more than offset by an increase in hospitalization costs.

[13]L. Breslow, "Changing Patterns of Medical Care and Support," *J. Med. Educ.* 41:318–324, 1966.

Additional References on Preventive Medicine

[1] *Proposed Preventive Benefits to be Covered on a First Dollar Basis Under National Health Insurance*, The American Public Health Association, July 16, 1974.

Lists a minimum set of preventive services and the frequency with which they should be offered under a first dollar basis under NHI (cost sharing is not desirable as it may encourage underutilization of preventive services). Underlying principles to assure their universal acceptability, high quality, and responsiveness are presented: (a) NHI payments should be made to agencies as well as individuals; (b) payments should include services provided by all members of the health team (not just physicians and dentists); (c) populations for whom preventive services are not available must be identified and provision made for their availability; and (d) minimum standards of quality must be established.

[2] *Incorporation of Preventive Medical Services into National Health Insurance*, a paper prepared for the Office of Management and Budget by Lester Breslow on behalf of the Association of Schools of Public Health and the Association of Teachers of Preventive Medicine, Nov. 19, 1973.

It is proposed that preventive medical services "packages," broken down by age and sex, be incorporated into national health insurance. A general rationale is presented for the development of a health-maintenance attitude on the part of both physician and patient rather than the complaint-response attitude typical of physicians and patients in the past.

[3] *Preventive Medical Services for National Health Insurance.* Report of a Fogarty International Center Task Force prepared under the auspices of the Office of the Assistant Secretary for Health, DHEW, May, 1974.

Proposals are presented in the form of specific preventive service packages applicable at different periods of life. The services which may be incorporated into National Health Insurance include those with clearly demonstrable benefit, approved by experts in the applicable field and generally accepted by the medical profession.

[4] J.M.G. Wilson and G. Jungner, *Principles and Practice of Screening for Disease*, Public Health Papers No. 34, Geneva, WHO, 1968, pp. 26–27.

[5] T. McKeown, "Validation of Screening Procedures," in *Screening in Medical Care*, London, Oxford University Press, 1968, pp. 1–13.

Presents comprehensive guidelines for evaluation of screening procedures.

[6] *Mass Health Examination as a Public Health Tool*, Technical Report No. A24, Geneva, WHO, 1971, pp. 50–51.

[7] A.L. Cochrane and W.W. Holland, "Validation of Screening Procedures," *Br. Med. Bull.* 25:3–8, 1971.

[8] L.G. Whitby, "Screening for Disease: Definitions and Criteria," *Lancet* 2:819–821, 1974.

[9] K.L. White, *Prevention as a National Goal* (Unpublished paper) 1974.

Three approaches to disease prevention are identified: containment, amelioration or cure of clinical disease, and screening and primary prevention. It is noted that to declare prevention of disease as a national health goal we must clearly state what is to be prevented, how and by whom.

[10] S. Waldman, *Preventive Service Under Major NHI Proposals* (DHEW unpublished paper) Dec. 2, 1974.

A summary of coverage of preventive services (physical exams, well-child care, prenatal and maternity care, family planning, vision exams, hearing exams, dental exams) under selected national health insurance proposals.

[11] D. Cardus (Editorial), "Towards a Medicine Based on the Concept of Health," *Prev. Med.* 2:309–312, 1973.

Emphasizes the need for a concept of health rather than disease.

[12] L. Breslow, *Health Maintenance: Personal Versus Social Responsibility*, Paper presented at meeting of the Practice Division of AAAS, June 19, 1974.

Discusses changes necessary to move toward a concept of health maintenance.

[13] Commission on Chronic Illness, *Chronic Illness in the United States Vol. I: Prevention of Chronic Illness*, Cambridge, Massachusetts, Harvard University Press, 1957.

[14] T. McKeown and E.G. Knox, "The Framework Required for Validation of Prescriptive Screening," in T. McKeown (ed.), *Screening in Medical Care*, London, Oxford University Press, 1968, pp. 159–170.

An assessment of what is required to adequately validate various screening procedures is presented.

[15] W.A. Krehl, "Prospective Medicine and the Compleat Physician," in L.C. Robbins (ed.), *Prospective Medicine and Health Hazard Appraisal*, Methodist Hospital of Indiana, 1974, pp. 1–6.

[16] L.C. Robbins, "The Prospective Model," in L.C. Robbins (ed.), *Prospective Medicine and Health Hazard Appraisal*, Methodist Hospital of Indiana, 1974, pp. 7–11.

[17] W.W. Holland, "Screening for Disease: Taking Stock," *Lancet* 2:1494–1497, 1974.

[18] K.M. Laurence, "Screening for Disease: Fetal Malformations and Abnormalities," *Lancet* 2:939–941, 1974.

[19] K.S. Holt, "Screening for Disease: Infancy and Childhood," *Lancet* 2:1057–1060, 1974.

[20] D.N. Raine, "Screening for Disease: Inherited Metabolic Disease," *Lancet* 2:996–998, 1974.

[21] T. Chard, "Screening for Disease: The Fetus at Risk," *Lancet* 2:880–883, 1974.

Appendix I. Criteria for the Evaluation of Screening Procedures

Introduction

Sets of specific criteria for evaluation of screening procedures have been advanced by Wilson and Jungner,[1] McKeown,[2] the World Health Organization,[3] Cochrane and Holland,[4] and Whitby.[5] These criteria are presented here.

Principles of Early Disease Detection[1]

1. The condition being sought should be an important health problem, for the individual and the community.
2. There should be an acceptable form of treatment for patients with recognizable disease.
3. The natural history of the condition, including its development from latent to declared disease, should be adequately understood.
4. There should be a recognizable latent or early symptomatic stage.
5. There should be a suitable screening test or examination for detecting the disease at the latent or early symptomatic stage, and this test should be acceptable to the population.
6. The facilities required for diagnosis and treatment of patients revealed by the screening programme should be available.
7. There should be an agreed policy on whom to treat as patients.
8. Treatment at the presymptomatic, borderline stage of a disease should favorably influence its course and prognosis.
9. The cost of case finding (which would include the cost of diagnosis and treatment) needs to be economically balanced in relation to possible expenditure on medical care as a whole.
10. Case finding should be a continuing process, not a "once and for all" project.

Criteria For Evaluation of Screening Procedures[2]

A. Definition of the problem
   1. What abnormality of medical significance is to be predicted or detected?

2. What prevention or therapy is to be offered?
3. Which group(s) is to be screened?
4. At what stage(s) is detection aimed?
5. What investigation and tests are proposed?
B. Review of position before screening
1. Evidence concerning the prevalence, natural history, and medical significance of the abnormality, with conclusions on the adequacy of the evidence.
2. Evidence concerning effectiveness of previous methods of preventing the disease.
3. Evidence concerning the effectiveness of previous methods of treating the disease.
C. Review of evidence concerning the screening procedure
1. Evidence concerning the effectiveness of the proposed diagnostic method(s).
   a. Applicability to group whose investigation is proposed;
   b. Error rates, positive and negative;
   c. Comparison with traditional diagnostic methods;
   d. Availability of resources;
   e. Acceptability;
   f. Cost;
   g. Conclusions on state of evidence on diagnostic method.
2. Evidence concerning the effectiveness of the proposed treatment.
   a. Applicability to group proposed;
   b. Comparison of effectiveness with treatment following conventional diagnosis;
   c. Availability of resources;
   d. Acceptability;
   e. Cost;
   f. Conclusions on state of evidence on treatment.
D. Conclusions concerning the state of evidence on the problem as a whole
1. Synthesis of evidence concerning natural history of the disease and the effects of the screening procedure as a whole, diagnosis and treatment being considered together.
2. Listing of medical gains and losses and comparison with similar balance sheets for alternative approaches to the problem.
3. Listing of financial costs and gains and comparison with alternative approaches.
E. Proposals for acquisition of further evidence
   Is further evidence necessary, and if so, what? What are the

logistics of the proposals and their relationship to available resources.

F. Proposals for initial applications

What application is justified? For what design, scale and duration should it be planned? How should it be supervised and what resources should be committed? Is the proposal mainly as a service on a research basis and if the latter, what information, or technical or operational developments, should be pursued?

Criteria for Evaluation of Screening Programs[3]

1. Screening must lead to an improvement in end results (defined in terms of mortality; physical, social, and emotional function; pain; and satisfaction) among those in whom early diagnosis is achieved or in the other members of the community.

   a. The therapy for the condition must favorably alter its natural history, not simply by advancing the point in time at which diagnosis occurs, but by improving survival, function, or both. The modification of "risk factors" is not sufficient evidence of effectiveness, nor is the fact that the proposed therapy is "commonly accepted." Claims for therapeutic effectiveness must withstand rigorous methodologic scrutiny, and experimental evidence, such as controlled clinical trials, is a prerequisite. The measurement of survival and other end results must withstand epidemiologic and biostatistical scrutiny.

   b. Available health services must be sufficient both to ensure diagnostic confirmation among those whose screening is positive and to provide long-term care.

   c. Compliance among asymptomatic patients in whom an early diagnosis has been achieved must be at a level to be effective in altering the natural history of the disease in question.

   d. The long-term beneficial effects, in terms of end results, must outweigh the long-term detrimental effects of the therapeutic regimen utilized and the "labeling" of an individual as "diseased" or "at high risk."

2. The effectiveness of potential components of multiphasic screening should be demonstrated individually prior to their combination.

3. If the benefits of screening accrue to the community at large rather than, or in addition to, the individual identified (e.g., disease carriers, specific occupations), the community benefit claimed must withstand scientific scrutiny.

a. The appropriateness of the mix of screening tests to the target population must be considered, acknowledging that differences in the distributions of two diseases may render the combination of their respective screening tests inappropriate.
4. The cost benefit and cost effectiveness characteristics of mass screening and long-term therapy must be known. This knowledge is considered essential in developing an appropriate mix of diagnostic and therapeutic services in the face of finite manpower and financial resources. Therefore, a mechanism for the formal periodic weighing of costs against benefits or effectiveness should constitute a basic component of the initial screening activities.
5. The burden of disability for the condition in question (in terms of disease frequency, distribution, severity, and alternative approaches to its detection and control) must warrant action.
6. The cost, sensitivity, specificity, and acceptability of the screening test must be known, and it should lend itself to the utilization patterns of the target population.
7. Ideally, an estimate of the social benefit of preventing, arresting, or curing the condition in question should be known.

Validation of Screening Test Methods[4]

1. *Simplicity.* In many screening programs more than one test is used to detect one disease, and in a multiphasic program the individual will be subjected to a number of tests within a short space of time. It is therefore essential that the tests used should be easy to administer and should be capable of use by paramedical and other personnel.
2. *Acceptabilty.* As screening is in most instances voluntary and a high rate of cooperation is necessary in an efficient screening programme, it is important that tests should be acceptable to the subjects.
3. *Accuracy.* The test should give a true measurement of the attribute under investigation.
4. *Cost.* The expense of screening should be considered in relation to the benefits resulting from the early detection of disease, i.e., the severity of the disease, the advantages of treatment at an early stage and the probability of cure.
5. *Precision* (sometimes called repeatability). The test should give consistent results in repeated trials.
6. *Sensitivity.* This may be defined as the ability of the test to give a positive finding when the individual screened has the disease or abnormality under investigation.

7. *Specificity*. This may be defined as the ability of the test to give a negative finding when the individual does not have the disease or abnormality under investigation.

Questions for Evaluation of Screening Procedures[5]

1. Is each abnormality that is being sought adequately defined (e.g., hypertension, hyperglycemia)?
2. What is considered to be the appropriate population to screen for the abnormality, and what is the basis for this selection?
3. Have epidemiological studies been carried out to establish the incidence or prevalence of the condition in a group similar to the one selected for screening, to serve as a basis for determining the validity (in terms of sensitivity and specificity) of the screening procedure in detecting abnormalities?
4. What screening methods are available and how do they compare with one another in acceptability, efficiency, and cost? Which seems to be the method of choice?
5. Are diagnostic facilities available for the follow-up of abnormalities revealed by the screening procedure, and is there an acceptable form of treatment for each condition revealed?
6. Have suitably controlled investigations been carried out to show that the natural history of the disease is favourably influenced by screening procedures, with their consequent possibility of early institution of treatment, as compared with allowing patients to present with the illness when symptoms demand attention?
7. What are the implications in terms of resources (education of the public, availability of staff, operating costs) of introducing, on a large scale, a screening program which has been shown to be worthwhile in a pilot study, and what difficulties are envisaged in moving from essentially a research investigation to routine everyday practice?
8. What is to be done about findings which are neither clearly normal nor obviously abnormal (the "borderline" problem)?

References

[1] J.M.G. Wilson and G. Jungner, *Principles and Practice of Screening for Disease*, Public Health Papers No. 34, Geneva, WHO, 1968, pp. 26–27.

[2] T. McKeown, "Validation of Screening Procedures, in *Screening in Medical Care*," London, Oxford University Press, 1968, pp. 1–13.

[3] *Mass Health Examination as a Public Health Tool*, Technical Report No. A24, Geneva, WHO, 1971, pp. 50–51.

[4] A.L. Cochrane and W.W. Holland, "Validation of Screening Procedures," *Br. Med. Bull.* 25:3–8, 1971.

[5] L.G. Whitby, "Screening for Disease: Definitions and Criteria," *Lancet* 2:819–821, 1974.

Appendix II. Preventive Medical Services Packages for National Health Insurance

Introduction

Preventive medical services can be incorporated into National Health Insurance by establishing "packages" of services to be provided at different periods of life. Three preventive medicine packages proposed for inclusion in National Health Insurance are presented below. These packages have been developed on behalf of the American Public Health Association, the Association of Schools of Public Health and the Association of Teachers of Preventive Medicine, and the Fogarty International Center.

Proposed Preventive Services

Proposed Preventive Benefits to be Covered on a First Dollar Basis Under National Health Insurance. The American Public Health Association, July 16, 1974.

I. Maternity Care
A. *Prenatal services*
The first visit, irrespective of when it occurs, should include the following components:

Health history
Physical examination
Laboratory examinations:
1. complete urinalysis
2. complete blood count
3. serological examination
4. chest x-ray
5. blood grouping and Rh determination, for both mother and father

6. cytology screening for genital tract malignancy

7. G.C. Culture

Subsequent visits should occur:

Once each month, through 28th week of pregnancy

Once each two weeks, 28-36 weeks of pregnancy

Once each week after 36th week of pregnancy

Laboratory tests for subsequent visits should include:

At each visit—urinalysis

In ninth month—also hemoglobin or hematocrit

During pregnancy, medication provided on a first dollar basis should include: routine vitamin and iron supplements.

Also, during this period, either group or individual instruction should be offered on nutrition, family planning, self-care, delivery and parenthood: up to 6 hours of group instruction each, for mother and father.

One home visit by a public health nurse, or other qualified health provider, for purposes of preparing the home and family for the absence of the mother during confinement, and for the care of the infant afterwards.

B. *Intrapartum Care*

All institutional and professional services associated with admission into an accredited hospital for purposes of giving birth, including managing labor, delivery, immediate postpartum care of the mother and newborn, including infantile resuscitation if necessary, routine care of the eyes and cord, testing for congenital diseases such as P.K.U., infantile serological testing, and care of the mother and baby in the hospital *through the fifth postpartum day*. Also, including costs of group or individual, supervised bedside instruction to the mother up to six hours total on self-care and infant care, and family planning. Too often, women, because of inadequate financial resources, are forced to leave the hospital too early without sufficient rest, knowledge of child care, and the benefit of family planning services. Also, during this immediate postpartum period, possible and potential problems with the infant can be identified.

C. *Postpartum Care*

One home visit by a public health nurse, or other qualified health provider, within the first two weeks after discharge from the hospital in order to assist with implementation of home care and to provide additional education for parenthood.

One office or clinic visit each for the mother and infant to their respective physicians during the first 8 weeks of the infant's life for routine examination, advisement, and laboratory procedures to include hemoglobin and urinalysis if they are indicated, and follow-up family planning services.

II. Preventive Child Care
  A. 1st year of life—seven visits
     2nd year of life—three visits
     3–6 years—one visit each year

     Included in these visits would be physical and laboratory examination, developmental evaluation, and immunization; as well as counseling and anticipatory guidance regarding nutrition, accidents, hygiene, and child development according to standards to be established by the Secretary of HEW.

  B. *6–18 Years*—Total costs of no more than one visit per year to an office or clinic for purposes of maintaining immunizations or for physical and/or developmental evaluations including necessary laboratory cost of first visits, and counseling regarding sexual development, alcoholism and drug abuse; and including five consultation visits when requests for those visits originate from a school health service for reasons of unsatisfactory progress in school.

  C. *Other Services*
     1. Routine dental services up to age 13 including: oral examination, x-ray, prophylaxis, topical fluoride application, counseling and education; and restorations including fillings, space maintenance, and extractions of deciduous teeth.
     2. Developmental vision care services up to age 18: routine eye examinations and provision of eyeglasses.
     3. Hearing: audiometry and provision of hearing aids up to age 18.

III. Adult Preventive Care (Male and Female)
   The following are basic preventive services for adults and the frequency with which they should be received. Specific preventive services for the female during the reproductive years are covered subsequent to this section.

   A. Between ages 18–30, two routine physicals (although more visits might be desirable, it is assumed that, during this period, the individual will receive additional physical examinations related to school, employment, and insurance).

   Between ages 31–40, three routine physicals

Between ages 41–50, four routine physicals
Between ages 51–60, five routine physicals
Over 60, an annual physical

All routine physical examinations should include general history; examination of heart, lungs, and abdomen; a rectal examination, complete blood count, urinalysis, chest x-ray; and, at least once every 10 years, screening for syphilis.

Above the age of 35, the general population is particularly at risk for certain specific problems. Thus, additional preventive screening measures should be performed as part of a routine physical examination. The problem areas and some of the tests for them include, but are not limited to:

1. *Cardiovascular problems*
   Tests should include blood pressure check for hypertension; a lipid profile, both for cholesterol and triglycerides; and an electrocardiogram.

2. *Gastrointestinal and prostate cancer*
   Including test for hidden blood in stool (stool guaiac), complete rectal examination, and sigmoidoscopy.

3. *Kidney disease*
   Tests should include chemistries for B.U.N. and creatinine; and urinalysis.

4. *Chest including lung cancer, emphysema, bronchitis, T.B., and cardiac problems*
   Tests include chest x-ray, tuberculin test, and screening pulmonary function tests (spirometry).

5. *Glaucoma*
   Tonometry

B. *Female Reproductive Care*
   In addition to the above preventive services, all women within the reproductive ages should receive, on an annual basis, breast and pelvic examinations, a Papanicolaou smear and a G.C. culture. The annual visit may also include health education, family planning counseling and provision of contraception (including pills), when prescribed, at no cost to the patient.

C. *Immunization*
   In accordance with the recommendations of a group designated by the Secretary (possibly within the Center for Disease Control) regarding the efficacy of specific immunizations, these shall be made available, when needed, on a first dollar basis for the adult population. These might include polio vaccine, gamma globulin, and flu shots.

D. *Routine Prophylaxis*

For certain at-risk groups within the population, routine prophylaxis has a known value in preventing medical catastrophe and in reducing hospitalization. Two specific prophylactic measures that should be included on a first dollar basis are regular penicillin for children with a history of rheumatic heart disease, and antibiotics for sufferers of cystic fibrosis. The application of other prophylactic techniques should also be included as they are recommended by a group designated by the Secretary (possibly located within the Center for Disease Control).

IV. Chronic Illness

A. Prevention programs for the chronically ill must be developed to meet two basic objectives:

1. Assist in the rehabilitation of a patient or reduce the possibility of further deterioration.

2. Prevent the need for high-cost hospitalization or other institutionalization; or, where hospitalization has already occurred, reduce the length of stay in an institutional setting and the danger of returning the individual to a facility.

B. Home health services are preventive not only in regard to reducing the amount and degree of morbidity, but as a true, low-cost alternative to expensive institutionalization. Limitations placed on these services, either through cost-sharing, or through restricting their utilization are, in our opinion, counter-productive: rather than representing a cost savings, they result in forcing the individual to remain in an institution for a longer period of time or to seek institutional services unnecessarily. Home health services, then, should be reimbursed by national health insurance when recommended by an evaluating professional (physician or nurse) as an alternative to potential or present hospitalization and should be given in accordance with a specific plan of treatment developed by a physician. The services should be offered through an accredited body that can provide a wide range of home health services including:

1. Skilled and nonskilled nursing care

2. Homemaking services

3. Social services

4. Physical and occupational therapy

5. Health and nutrition education to both the patient and the family

V. Health Education
Health education benefits should be geared to meet the following objectives for the population:
A. Development of appropriate self-management techniques and the assurance that an individual is complying with a prescribed regimen.
B. Assistance to health consumer to utilize benefits appropriately.
C. Mitigation of risks leading to health problems, the minimization of the effects of an illness, and avoidance of its recurrence.
D. Orientation of the individual to seek early screening or treatment and towards changing patterns of health behavior.

Health education benefits should be provided to the consumer in a variety of settings where health education is an integral, continuous component of any organized comprehensive health delivery system, and should be offered on both an individual and small group basis. Services should be available with such programs as HMOs, hospitals, neighborhood health centers, schools, and industrial settings.

The specific types of health education activities proposed include:
1. General preventive efforts, e.g., smoking reduction, weight control, exercise, nutrition, VD education, and changing health behavior patterns.
2. Specific highly targeted programs, to groups either at risk for, or who already have a disease condition, e.g., hypertension control, pregnancy, or maintenance of diabetic regimen.

These services are to be reimbursable when they are offered by qualified health education personnel and are *in addition* to standard physician/nurse-patient therapeutic encounters. Health education services which include the use of pamphlets or audiovisual devices without the direct intervention of trained health education personnel are not to be covered.

Proposed Preventive Services

Incorporation of Preventive Medical Services into National Health Insurance. A paper prepared for the Office of Management and Budget by Lester Breslow on behalf of the Association of Schools of Public Health and the Association of Teachers of Preventive Medicine, November 19, 1973.

AGE	*PROCEDURES*

I. Mother and fetus
   Prenatal care

Prenatal history
Examination, including:
   Height, weight
   Urine-sugar and albumen
   VDRL
   Blood pressure
   Blood typing

Counseling, regarding:
   Nutrition
   Cigarette smoking
   Delivery

II. Birth to One Year
   A. Normal infant care

Four visits to physician or physician-supervised assistant for observation and measurement of growth and development, including:
   Complete immunization schedule

Parent counseling (and other measures) to assure necessary follow-up of abnormalities, and regarding:
   Nutrition
   Hygiene
   Behavior
   Accidents

   B. High-risk infant

Six visits (otherwise same as under IIA)

III. 5–6 Years
   School entry assessment

Review and completion of immunization schedule.

Review of health systems, with particular reference to:
   Vision
   Hearing
   Speech
   Teeth
   Urine culture (females)
   Urine sugar and albumen

Parent, child, and teacher counseling (and other measures) needed for follow-up, and regarding:
   Nutrition
   Accidents

IV. 12–14 Years
   Puberty assessment

Immunization review and booster

Growth and systems review Examination, including:
   Skin
   Teeth

91

Blood pressure
Vision
Hearing
Urine culture (females)
Urine sugar and albumen

Counseling regarding:
Sexual development, including
contraception and venereal disease
Nutrition
Cigarettes, alcohol, drugs
Accidents (emphasis on safe driving)

V. 17–19 Years
    Adult entry assessment

Examination including:
Height, weight
Blood pressure
Blood cholesterol
Vision, hearing, teeth
VDRL
Culture for gonorrhea
(females only)
Urine sugar and albumen

Counseling regarding:
Family planning, including
genetic problems
Cigarettes, alcohol, drugs
Nutrition
Exercise
Accidents

VI. 24–26 Years and Every
    5 Years Till Age 44
      Young adult assessment

Examination including:
Height, weight
Blood pressure
Blood cholesterol
Urine sugar and albumen
Papanicolaou smear
(females)

Counseling regarding:
Cigarettes, alcohol, drugs
Nutrition
Exercise
Sleep

VII. 45–46 Years and Every
    5 Years Till Age 59
      Middle-age assessment

Examination including:
Height, weight
Blood pressure
Blood cholesterol
Blood sugar

92

                    EKG
                    Papanicolaou smear
                    (females)
                    Breast, including
                    Mammography (females)
                    Vision and tonometry
                    Blood in stool
                    Rectal

                    Counseling regarding:
                    Cigarettes, alcohol, drugs
                    Nutrition
                    Exercise
                    Sleep

VIII. 59–61 Years and Every
      2 Years Thereafter
      Older-age assessment

                    Examination including:
                    Height, weight
                    Blood pressure
                    Blood sugar
                    EKG
                    Mammography (females)
                    Papanicolaou smear
                    (females)
                    Vision and tonometry
                    Hearing
                    Blood in stool
                    Rectal

                    Counseling, regarding:
                    Nutrition
                    Alcohol and drugs
                    Exercise
                    Sleep
                    Retirement plans

Proposed Preventive Services

Preventive Medical Services for National Health Insurance. Report of a Fogarty International Center Task Force prepared under the auspices of the Office of the Assistant Secretary for Health, DHEW, May 1974.

Table 1. Maternity Package

STAGE OF PREGNANCY	PREGNANCY DIAGNOSIS	1st TRIMESTER	2nd TRIMESTER	3rd TRIMESTER	DELIVERY	POST-NATAL	COMMENTS
Number of Visits	1-4 per Annum	3	3	8	5	1	
Measurements							
Weight		X	X	X	X	X	
BP		X	X	X	X	X	
Uterine Size		X	X	X	X	X	
Temperature					X		
Assessments							
Risk Assessment	X						Determination of risk at earliest stage possible—
Progress of Pregnancy			X	X			
Interval History		X	X	X		X	
Review: Preg-Delivery		X	X	X	X	X	
Physical Exam.		X			X		Complete physical examination only on initial visit; subsequent PE as indicated
Dental Exam.		X					
Screening Tests							Complete battery of screening procedures on initial visit only. Biochemical profile—SMA12 To include: blood glucose creatinine SGOT calcium serum proteins
HI-Gonadotropin	X						
Hemoglobin-Hematocrit		X	X	X	X		
Blood Group-Rh		X					
Father Typed		X					
Blood Smear	X	X					
Rubella Antibody	X	X					
Au Antigen		X					
Tuberculin		X					
VDRL		X					
Gonococcal Culture						X	
Pap Smear			X			X	
Urinalysis		X	X	X	X		

Procedure / Counseling				Notes
Biochem: Profile	X			
Procedures				
Immunization				
Tetanus	X			X*
TOPY				X*
Rubella				X*
Amniocentesis	X	X		
Gamma globulin	X	X		
Anti-Rh Titers	X	X		
Cephalometry				
Urinary Estrogen/Creatinine				
Tachodynamometry		X		
Urine culture		X		
Urinary Urea N/Total N		X		
Counseling				
Advantage of early diagnosis	X	X		
Contraception	X	X		
Family Planning		X		
Risks to Developing Fetus	X			
Disorders of Early Pregnancy	X			
Nutrition	X			
Smoking	X			
Abortion	X			
Congenital Anomalies	X			
Physiology of Labor				
Delivery	X			
Infant Care	X			

* Special procedures apply to 2nd and 3rd trimesters only if needed based on risk assessment

Counseling format where applicable throughout the course of pregnancy and postnatal period

Table 2. Child and Adolescent Packages

AGE	BIRTH	1-6 MOS.	7-17 MOS.	1½-4 YRS.	SCHOOL ENTRY 5-6 YRS.	EARLY ADOLESCENCE 11-13 YRS.	ADULT ENTRY 17-19 YRS.
Number of Visits	*1*	*3-4*	*3-5*	*4*	*2-3*	*2-3*	*2-3*
Measurements							
Height	X	X	X	X	X	X	X
Weight	X	X	X	X	X	X	X
Head Circumference	X	X					
B. P.					X(2)[d]	X(2)[d]	X(2)[d]
Assessments							
Development	X[a]	X	X	X	X		X
Interval History		X	X	X	X	X(1)	X
Behavior					X		
Physical Examination	X	X(1)[c]	X(1)[c]		X(1)[c]	X(1)[b,c]	X(1)[c]
Dental Examination					X(1)[c]	X(0)[c]	
Screening Tests (One per age group)							
Vision	X	X		X	X	X	X
Hearing	X	X		X	X		X
Speech				X	X		
Tuberculin			X	X	X	X	X
PKU	X						
Hemoglobin/Hematocrit			X	X	X	X	X
Urinalysis				X	X	X	X
Urine Culture (f)					X(2)[d]	X(2)[d]	X(2)[d]
Sickle Cell Trait						X	Other Lab Tests: VDRL, G.C. cult. Cholesterol
Special Procedures							
Immunizations DTP Polio Measles Mumps Rubella	DTP TOPV	DTP TOPV	Measles Mumps Rubella		DTP TOPV	Rubella[e]	Td booster Rubella[e]

96

Counseling:						
Feeding	X					
Use of H M Service	X					
Use of Care Service	X					
Immunizations						
Nutrition	X	X				
Accidents	X	X		X		
Poisons	X	X				
Oral Hygiene				X	X	
Smoking				X		X
Sex Hygiene				X		X
Contraception					X	X
Drugs					X	X
Alcohol					X	X

[a] Review of pregnancy and delivery history; review Apgar scores.

[b] Including sexual development.

[c] Required only once during the age indicated.

[d] Required only twice during the age indicated.

[e] Recommended for females during these age periods.

[f] Counseling format is adjusted to age group; subject coverage may be repetitive and cumulative in attempt to reinforce life style guidelines.

Table 3. Young Adult Package

AGE GROUPS: 24-26, 29-31, 34-36 SCHEDULE: One visit per age group or three visits minimum during period 24-36	NO. VISITS	MEASURE- MENTS	ASSESS- MENTS	PHYSICAL EXAM.	SCREENING	SPECIAL PROCE- DURES	COUNSEL- ING	REFERRAL SEQUENCE
Procedures								
Immunizations	1					X		
Height, Weight	1	X					X	Rx
Blood Pressure	2			X			X	
EKG	1[a]				X			Dx[b]
Blood Chemistries								
Cholesterol					X			
Triglycerides					X			
Glucose					X			
Uric Acid					X			
SGOT					X			
Other Laboratory Procedures	1[a]							
Hemoglobin					X			Dx[b]
Urinalysis					X			Dx[b]
Cervical Smear- Carcinoma	1				X			Dx[b]
History/Life Style Review	1							
Headache			X					Dx[b]
Chest Pain			X					
Urinary Symptoms			X					Dx[b]
Bowel Habit			X					Dx[b]
Bleeding			X					
Smoking							X	
Alcohol							X	

[a] Abnormal value is regarded as presumptive evidence of disease state and requires confirmation; additional diagnostic procedures may be indicated. With computer controlled automated systems, a second visit may not be required.

[b] Dx Abnormal finding requires diagnostic follow-up with one additional visit in preventive services package.

Table 4. Middle-Age Package

AGE GROUPS:
40-46, 50-52, 55-57
SCHEDULE: One visit per age group or three visits minimum during period
40-57

	NO. VISITS	MEASURE-MENTS	ASSESS-MENTS	PHYSICAL EXAM.	SCREENING	SPECIAL PROCE-DURES	COUNSEL-ING	REFERRAL SEQUENCE
Procedures								
Immunizations	1							
Height, Weight	1	X						
Blood Pressure	2					X	X	Rx
EKG	1a			X			X	Dx^b
Blood Chemistries								
Cholesterol					X			
Triglycerides					X			
Glucose					X			
Uric Acid					X			
SGOT					X			
Other Laboratory Procedures	1							
Hemoglobin					X			Dx^b
Stool Guaiac					X			Dx^b
Urinalysis	1				X			Dx^b
Tonometry-Glaucoma	1				X			Dx^b
Cervical Smear-Carcinoma	1				X			Rx^b
Mammography	1				X			Dx^b
History/Life Style Review	1							Dx^b
Headache			X					
Chest Pain			X					
Urinary Symptoms			X					Dx^b
Bowel Habit			X					
Bleeding			X					Dx^b
Smoking			X					Dx^b
Alcohol			X				X	

a Abnormal value is regarded as presumptive evidence of disease state and requires confirmation; additional diagnostic procedures may be indicated. With computer controlled automated systems, a second visit may not be required.

b Dx Abnormal finding requires diagnostic follow-up with one additional visit in preventive services package.

Table 5. Older Adult Package

AGE GROUPS: 60 AND >60 SCHEDULE: One visit every five years	NO. VISITS	MEASUREMENTS	ASSESSMENTS	PHYSICAL EXAM.	SCREENING	SPECIAL PROCEDURES	COUNSELING	REFERRAL SEQUENCE
Procedures								
Immunizations						X	X	Rx
Height, Weight		X					X	
Blood Pressure				X	X		X	
EKG								
Vision		X						
Hearing	1[a]	X						Dx[b]
Blood Chemistries								
Cholesterol					X			
Triglycerides					X			
Glucose					X			
Uric Acid					X			
SGOT					X			
Other Laboratory	1[a]							
Procedures								
Hemoglobin					X			Dx[b]
Stool Guaiac					X			Dx[b]
Urinalysis								Dx[b]
Cervical Smear-Carcinoma	1				X			Dx[b]
Physical Examinations								
Breast				X				
Rectal-prostate				X				
Podiatry				X				
Dental				X				
History/Life Style Review	1							
Headache			X					Dx[b]
Chest Pain			X					
Urinary Symptoms			X					

Bowel Habit	X	Dx[b]
Bleeding	X	Dx[b]
Smoking	X	X
Alcohol	X	X
Nutrition	X	X
Housing	X	X
Social Habits	X	

[a]Abnormal value is regarded as presumptive evidence of disease state and requires confirmation; additional diagnostic procedures may be indicated. With computer controlled automated systems, a second visit may not be required.

[b]Dx Abnormal finding requires diagnostic follow-up with one additional visit in preventive services package.

Task Force Members

Mildred A. Morehead, M.D., M.P.H., *Chairman*
Director, Evaluation Unit
Associate Professor
Department of Community Health
Albert Einstein College
  of Medicine
Bronx, New York

Paul M. Densen, D.SC.
Director
Center for Community Health
  and Medical Care
Boston, Massachusetts

Mary E.W. Goss, PH.D.
Professor of Sociology
  in Public Health
Cornell University
  Medical College
Department of Public Health
New York, New York

Ruth J. Helmich, C.N.M.
Research Associate
Evaluation Unit
Department of Community Health
Albert Einstein College
  of Medicine
Bronx, New York

Mr. Sam Shapiro
Health Services Research
  and Development Center
Johns Hopkins University
Baltimore, Maryland

Cecil Sheps, M.D.
Vice Chancellor
Health Sciences
University of North Carolina
Chapel Hill, North Carolina

Mr. Gerald Sparer
Acting Director
Division of Health Services Evaluation
DHEW—Public Health Service
Health Resources Administration
Rockville, Maryland

James Zimmer, M.D.
Associate Professor
Department of Preventive Medicine
  and Community Health
University of Rochester
Rochester, New York

I. Introduction

The evaluation of preventive health services and programs, as well as controls over the quality of the modalities utilized, is receiving increased attention by both the public and the health profession. Whether such efforts will be sustained in the face of a decreasing economy and with the ever increasing pressure of funds for direct service is problematic. Efforts to assure adequate standards and performance have lagged because of the lack of commitment to this programmatic component, inadequate funds, lack of mechanisms to enforce compliance and debate over the efficacy and relevance of the methods employed to achieve the desired objectives. In spite of these difficulties, however, there can be little rationale for the expenditure of vast sums of money, time, and resources without concomitant efforts to ensure that, as a minimum, there is application of standards of performance that can be accepted by the profession as the best available knowledge at this time.

Even though knowledge of many diseases is limited, techniques for measurement not all of proven value, and public and political pressure frequently the program determinant rather than need and rationality, it is essential that quality controls and evaluation be an integral part of any health program.

Primary prevention—the avoidance of disease, disability, and premature death, is increasingly difficult to effect in an era where chronic disease and individual behavior patterns are the causes of major public health problems. The breakthroughs that led to the control of the great scourges of communicable disease in the past have in large measure reduced these hazards. To adequately protect a population from diabetes, cancer, accidents, suicide, and to improve the living conditions of those more subject to disease by virtue of poverty and ignorance, requires new methods of prevention which will need assessment by sophisticated tools and measurements that are only minimally available or in the developmental stage at the present time.

Secondary prevention, the early detection of disease, slowing progression of pathology, preventing complications and disability while maximizing health status and functioning, has received proportionately more emphasis than primary prevention by the "curing" oriented health professions. It is in this area that the major thrust for evaluation and quality controls has arisen, e.g., peer review, cost efficiency, etc., even though here too, such efforts are not sufficiently widespread and are aimed more at cost containment than at the quality of service provided or on the impact of the care on the population served. Nevertheless, there are at hand considerably more approaches than are currently utilized to study, improve and effect change in the health delivery system. The deficiencies in methods and disagreements over effectiveness should not be permitted to stand as obstacles to the monitoring and review of current performance and programs to see that, as a minimum, adverse effects are not produced and as a maximum, that the best of the current body of scientific knowledge is applied to the greatest number of persons in ways that can benefit general health and living conditions. Implicit in this latter statement is examination not only of the efficacy of a program or provider but whether indeed programs exist and are adequately distributed to meet the nation's health requirements.

Periodic, systematic review of a community's health problems and needs with a recording of priorities when indicated is essential for adequate planning and introduction of appropriate elements of preventive health programs of all levels.

In recent years, there has been increasing emphasis by federal regulatory agencies as well as professional groups, on quality control, evaluation, and utilization of direct health services. In large measure, these have been responses to public concern over the quality of care and cost of medical care. In 1965, requirements for in-hospital utilization review were contained in the Medicare legislation (Title XVIII). The passage of PL 92-603, Professional Standards Review Organization (PSRO) in 1972 mandated professional review of the quality of care on a nationwide basis. Various professional organizations also have developed guidelines for quality assessment. The American Hospital Association also developed a guide for a Quality Assurance Program (QAP) which interrelated the utilization review program and the medical audit. And in 1973, the Joint Commission on Accreditation of Hospitals added a requirement to their accreditation process, i.e., "to become and remain accredited by the JCAH, a hospital now must demonstrate that it has an internal system of controls to assure the quality of care rendered to its patients"; the Performance Evaluation Procedure (PEP) was developed as a guide. Numerous other medical societies (e.g., New York State Hospital Utilization Review Superior Method [NYSHUR], New Jersey's Approval by Individual Diagnosis [AID]), Blue Cross agencies as well as national and regional data systems such as the Professional Activities Study (PAS and MAP) which have been active for several decades, are active in current efforts.

Review of the functions, financing and both internal and external controls of these organizations was considered beyond the scope of this Task Force as their major emphasis relates to cost and quality of curative services rather than preventive services. The committee urges, however, that as further experience is gained through these efforts, attention be given to the inclusion of preventive health modalities as an area which would have equal, if not greater, long-range impact on the nation's health.

In summary, this Task Force has taken the position that *there should be assessment of the adequacy of the prevalence of preventive health programs and providers and that the objectives and standards of performance of a program or a provider should be clearly enumerated. Such standards and objectives should then be periodically and systematically evaluated to assure that goals are met. Concomitantly, there should be continued application of quality controls and evaluation of standards to assure that the most effective modalities are employed to impact on the nation's health. In order to assure that these objectives are obtained, a public commitment supported by adequate program policies and funding is required.*

To examine any health care program, standards and objectives should be set for each of the following areas (Table 1) for both primary and secondary preventive health activities and evaluation and quality controls operative at each step.

Table 1. Matrix for Evaluation

PREVENTIVE MEDICINE IS THAT BRANCH OF MEDICINE WHICH HAS PRIMARY INTEREST IN:

SECONDARY PREVENTION

PRIMARY PREVENTION

SLOWING THE PROGRESS OF DISEASE AND CONSERVING MAXIMAL FUNCTION[a]

PREVENTING PHYSICAL, MENTAL AND EMOTIONAL DISEASE AND INJURY IN CONTRAST TO TREATING THE SICK AND INJURED

ELEMENTS OF A PREVENTIVE HEALTH PROGRAM (PERSONAL AND ENVIRONMENTAL HEALTH)

Element	Example from Secondary Prevention	Example from Primary Prevention
Program Objective	Early detection of disease, maximize health status, prevention of complications	Environmental hazards, behavior modification, reduction of protection from communicable disease
Structure and Organization	Private physician, nurse practitioner	Health Department, school system, voluntary agency, group practice
Clinical Modality	Adequate data base, appropriate therapy	Immunizations
Laboratory Modality	Monitoring of blood sugars, BUNs	Pap smears, lead levels, hemoglobins, chest x-rays
Health Education Modality	Compliance with medication regime, weight reduction	Smoking, accident prevention

EVALUATION OF PREVENTIVE HEALTH PROGRAMS
(PERSONAL AND ENVIRONMENTAL HEALTH)

Evaluation Element	Example from Secondary Prevention	Example from Primary Prevention
Penetration Rate	Proportion of target population with disease or condition under ongoing care	Proportion of target population reached
Cost Efficiency	Unit cost per newly discovered case, per case of controlled disease	Unit cost for immunization, fluoridation
Structure and Organization	Facilities, staff, organization, financing, integration of programs; provider range of therapeutic services, follow-up	Facilities, staff, organization, financing, integration of programs; identification and analysis of primary preventive program
Process Measures Clinical	Review of clinical performance by implicit/explicit criteria, tracers	Adequate maintenance of immunizations
Laboratory	Appropriate studies performed	Assessment of quality controls and accuracy of studies
Health Education	Behavioral modification, patient compliance	Knowledge by the population, behavioral modification, accuracy and appeal of material and techniques
Program Result Measures Reduction of Incidence	Reduction of complications of disease or condition	Reduction of disease or condition
Health Status	Maximization of individual health status	Decreased mortality or morbidity, decreased work days lost

[a]American College of Preventive Medicine's definition of Preventive Medicine.

107

II. Evalution Methodologies

Penetration Rate

The basic definition is the proportion of a target population that is provided a service which by itself, or when followed by prescribed medical or behavioral activities, is expected to result (1) in the prevention of a disease or condition (primary prevention), or (2) in the detection of a disease or condition at a stage in which its course could be favorably altered (secondary prevention). In order to achieve maximum results or yield, the population or subset thereof that is at risk, should be clearly identified in relation to the anticipated effect of the modality or intervention to be utilized.

The target population in either primary or secondary preventive programs will vary depending upon several factors, including: (a) the organization and responsibilities of the preventive program sponsors; (b) the condition to be prevented and its at-risk population; (c) the nature of the preventive procedure; and (d) basic program constraints such as available funds, legal and logistical considerations, etc. Target populations can be delineated by three main sets of characteristics:

1. Geographical (and/or political) boundary.

2. Eligibility for service; such as health program subscriber (enrollee) populations, benefit groups such as Medicaid and Veterans Administration, employee groups (identified by company, industry, civil service, military, school, etc.).

3. Populations based on special "opportunities" such as;
   a. the occurrence of a specific event, such as hospitalization or traffic violation, which led to the automatic institution of either a preventive screening activity or a health educational program (for example, the required cervical cancer screening of hospitalized women over the age of 20 or the required driving skills education classes held for drivers with multiple traffic violations);
   b. institutional residences (e.g., nursing homes, prisons); and
   c. use of clinic facilities in institutions, or ambulatory care through other primary care providers.

Each of these types of target population can be further defined or approached for a preventive service out of the total population eligible on the basis of either (a) total population by geography, subscription, etc., or (b) as a specific at-risk subgroup of that population which may be defined by demographic, exposure, and other characteristics.

In addition to the concern for the basic penetration rate in both primary and secondary preventive programs, an essential element of importance in the evaluation of such programs is an analysis of the "nonpenetrated" groups within the target population.

While the techniques to examine penetration rates may vary, clearly it is necessary to have a defined population against which any rate is to be measured. In the case of a prepaid group practice plan, this may be readily available for some limited population characteristics; for other population groups, it may be necessary to develop data based on a population census or on a random sample survey. The random sample survey, of course, has the advantage of including variables which may not have been asked in a census.

There are some methodological problems in obtaining the penetration rate. For example, in the HIP Mammography Study, information on participants was based on self-administered questionnaires and interviews conducted in person at the screening sites. Numerator information was based on mailed questionnaires and telephone interviews. Limited methodological research seems to indicate that the differences in responses obtained among these different methods are of only small importance in some subject areas.

The kinds of information which may be obtained are, of course, related to study purposes. The HIP breast cancer studies examined issues such as previous preventive health care behavior, involvement in the HIP medical care system, concern with cancer, and beliefs concerning the efficacy of screening procedures. Studies in immunization, however, should touch on other matters since primary prevention, rather than early detection, is the major focus.

The resulting information should enable comparisons to be made between participants and nonparticipants. In addition, if it is possible to obtain this comparison during the course of the study, it may permit changes in the approach to the target population which could improve the response and penetration rate. If it is found that the procedure in the preventive health program is thought by persons in the target population to involve pain, for example, and this is not the case, then the absence of pain might be mentioned in contacting the target population.

Analysis of data may be of significant usefulness in determining the bias among participants. There is consistent evidence that the better educated and those who tend to seek medical care also tend to participate in preventive health programs. It may be that the nonparticipants are involved in other health care systems which could be involved in the preventive health program. It may also be that self-selection occurs on a rational basis, i.e., those of greatest risk may tend to participate more than others. This could be a desirable occurrence.

Raymond Fink, Sam Shapiro, and John Lewison, "The Reluctant Participant in a Breast Cancer Screening Program," *Public Health Reports,* 6:479, 1968.

Raymond Fink, Sam Shapiro, Sidney S. Goldensohn, and Edwin F. Daily, "The 'Filter-Down' Process to Psychotherapy in a Group Practice Medical Care Program," *American Journal of Public Health,* 2:245, February 1969.

Raymond Fink, Sam Shapiro, and Ruth Roester, "Impact of Efforts to Increase Participation in Repetitive Screenings for Early Breast Cancer Detection," *American Journal of Public Health,* 62:328, March 1972.

Raymond Fink, Paper presented at Behavioral Sciences Conference sponsored by the National Cancer Institute, Division of Cancer Control and Rehabilitation, San Antonio, Texas, January 20, 1975.

Joann H. Langston et al., *Analysis of Relationships between Selected Organizational/Functional and Performance characteristics of OEO Neighborhood Health Centers,* Geomet Report No. SF-212, 1973.

System Sciences, Inc., *Comprehensive Health Services Project Data Base Report, Fourth Quarter, 1973.* Prepared for the Division of Monitoring and Analysis, Bureau of Community Health Services, DHEW, HSM 110-73-496, June 1974.

Cost Efficiency

The definition of efficiency for both primary and secondary prevention in general terms is the same, and is simply cost per unit of output. Efficiency measurement is not concerned with effects of the output units on persons or environment but only with the fact of the unit having been produced, and its cost. However, ideally the units of output should be adjusted in some way to include the concept of quality, i.e., a quality adjusted unit. Implicit in efficiency measurement is the assumption that there are comparable systems or alternative preventive programs with similar targets and goals, with which to compare the unit costs.

Evaluation of efficiency can be aimed in two directions; first, at the question of maximization of units of output for a fixed input, in other words, increasing output for a given total program cost; and second, at the reduction of input for each unit of output, that is, reducing the cost of each output unit.

Cost effectiveness analysis is an analytic approach in which the benefits of a given program are kept constant and the analyst determines the cost of alternative ways of generating those benefits: the assumption here would be that alternative programs really do generate the same benefits. One is not interested in finding out whether the program is worth doing at all (i.e., what is the most efficient way of treating end-stage kidney disease?).

110

Note, however, that in determining the most efficient way of producing a given level of output or in doing cost efficiency analysis in general, one needs to take four factors into consideration:

1. Is the quality of the output the same or can allowances be made in the analyses for differential quality?
2. Are there externalities, i.e., does this treatment have effects beyond the case under consideration?
3. Are there interactions among programs?
4. Are there economies of scale, i.e., does the cost per unit of output depend on the scale of the program?

The last is obviously of importance since the relative cost effectiveness of two programs may depend on where they are introduced.

Structure and Organization

The definition and delineation of the "structure" of a preventive service program is complex in that it is often an integral part of a larger health care provision entity; that is, one which provides curative, supportive, and rehabilitative services for acute and chronic illness. Also, preventive programs are often a part of health departments or the equivalent, where other types of activity are performed as well. There are, in fact, a variety of kinds of health care entities which have responsibility for initiating and conducting preventive programs; examples are health departments, school systems, organized care delivery systems, public, voluntary and private agencies, and individual providers. In evaluating the structure, and this is likewise relevant to the consideration of evaluating "process" (next section) of a preventive program, two general questions must be asked:

1. Is the structure of the preventive program *itself*, identified as well as possible within its parent system, appropriate and optimum as a framework for the "process" of providing the service? For example, are the organization, staff, facilities, etc., of a multiphasic screening program, which is run by an HMO, appropriate and effective for the screening program? And are the linkages with other components of the organization sufficiently defined to assure identification and follow-up of abnormal findings?

2. Is the structural *setting* of the preventive program appropriate and does it lead to optimum efficiency and effectiveness? For example, is an outpatient department setting and structure optimum for a family planning program, or should it be free-standing or related to some other entity? Or, is the structure a particular general pediatric group practice the optimum setting for provision of preventive services and well-child care, and are they appropriately integrated into the entire practice?

Evaluative techniques for assessment of "structure" are generally normative and criteria based, leading to the establishment of standards for organization, staff, qualifications, facilities, equipment, etc. "Normative" standards, however, should be accepted only until objective data support the standards utilized. As with "process," below, "structure" is an important element which determines system efficiency, and this can become one of the more objective evaluative measures.

One example of the areas to be examined in relation to structure and organization can be found in the federally supported evaluative efforts of the neighborhood health centers where certain areas are examined by combined normative and explicit criteria (Table 2).

Clinical Modalities

While efficiency is one overall measure of the "quality" of process, it is essential to look in greater detail at subsets of the process of providing preventive services. Since this kind of evaluation is directed at specific operational modalities within the system, it is usually, considering the state of the art, based on normative, or "expert opinion," criteria. These criteria, in turn, may have been derived from evidence of efficiency and efficacy of the types of operational modality being evaluated, but when applied to a particular preventive program, the criteria are accepted, as is, as the basis for standards against which characteristics of the operational modalities are measured. Thus, for example, certain standards of task performance time might be used, or repeatability (reliability) standards for laboratory tests [1,2] might be set, against which process performance is evaluated.

Primary Prevention

There are at the present time few clinical interventions that can prevent disease: immunizations, prophylactic gamma globulin in the face of infectious hepatitis contact, plaque removal for the prevention of caries and administration of RhoGAM in Rh-negative women are among the few instances that have demonstrated effectiveness.

Quality control of such modalities would entail seeing that the biological ingredients employed are standardized, free from contamination, and applied in a manner to achieve maximum body response.

Evaluation of such programs would require, in addition to determination of penetration rates, monitoring of results to see that objectives continue to meet, the collection of data regarding untoward reactions, weighed against the degree of infectiousness, e.g., rabies control.

As primary prevention moves from the field of infectious disease to

Table 2. Areas Reviewed in Neighborhood Health Centers [a,b]

Center Operations
  Target Area Community and Population;
    Center Accessibility
  Physical Facilities
Patient Flow
  Eligibility and Registration
  Appointment System
  Patient Acceptance
Administrative Services
  Program Management
  Business and Fiscal Administration
  Personnel Administration
  Program Analysis and Reporting
Medical Care Organization
Within the Center
  Family-Oriented Care
  Team Care
  Provider Staffing and Productivity
Medical Care Relationships Within the Community
  Backup Hospital Relationships
  Relationships With Other Health and Community Programs
Supportive Services
  Psychosocial Services
  Nursing Services
  Care by Middle-Level Practitioners
  Training and Utilization of New Health Workers
  Medical Records
  Transportation
  Laboratory
  Pharmacy
  Radiology
  Nutrition
  Physical Medicine and Rehabilitation
Community Participation and Consumer Involvement

[a]Excludes Quality of Health Services Reviews
[b]*Ambulatory Health Care Services Review Manual*, Evaluation Unit, Department of Community Health, Albert Einstein College of Meicine.

that of the chronic illness, controlled clinical trials of long duration will be necessary to determine, for example, whether changes in food content reduce the incidence of hypertension or diabetes.

While such large scale trials will be difficult to undertake, their usefulness in many conditions for primary prevention will be limited until such time as more exact scientific knowledge is available about the evolution (epidemiology) of specific diseases, their physiological cause and the nature of intervention that will avert onset of the condition.

Secondary Prevention

Evaluation of clinical performance and intervention to prevent complications and maximize health status rests upon a series of approaches which are currently being widely debated as to their efficacy and usefulness. As in any field of endeavor, when multiple methodologies are

113

being espoused to reach the same objective, one can be reasonably certain that there is no one clear-cut answer. Among the more common of the methods employed or proposed today are:

Process Measurement Process measurement is the systematic observation of what is done for and to a patient in light of current knowledge of disease and is generally based on peer consensus as to appropriate modalities. Such management can be based on retrospective chart review, observation of the provider, or repeat examination of the patient. Included among the process measurements are:

1. Implicit Peer Review

This approach rests on the clinical judgement of the reviewing physician who, subconsciously using his "mental computer," gathers facts from all aspects of a patient's problem, analyzes them into a unique whole for that individual, and assesses the adequacy of the course of action based on such analysis. This method rests to a considerable extent upon the skill and judgement of the reviewer and the extent to which his opinion is valued by his peers.[3-5]

The disadvantages of this approach are that it is time-consuming, expensive, and has been faulted for lack of objectivity and reproducibility. These latter two objections, of valid concern, rest in large measure on the degree of refinement that is sought. To distinguish excellence, for example, from good performance, will be subject to more disagreement than to distinguish unacceptable practice from optimal current standards. It will also depend upon the amount of agreement about clinical modalities. There will be more disagreement about immediate surgical intervention in subacute cholecystitis than for appendicitis.

The degree of control or structure of the study design also affects the degree of reproducibility. The studies conducted by the New York State Bureau of Medical Review, reported from a study of 1,258 complicated obstetrical cases in the Rochester Hospital Service Region, revealed more variation in expert opinion than had been expected; the proportion of final judgement disagreements was found to be 33 percent.[6] On the other hand, where reviewers met to discuss their findings, or instructions were fairly well structured, disagreements were far lower.[7,8]

Another disadvantage is logistical in that the review can only be conducted on small samples since the availability of experts for this is limited, and not all physicians, irrespective of their eminence or degree of integrity, make good reviewers. To be able to summarize and analyze given case materials takes a skill that is rather elusive to define.

The advantages of this approach are that it can take into account the variations in reaction of individual patients, both physiological and psychological, as well as the presence of concomitant disease which is

114

frequently the most important determinant of the patient's eventual health status.

2. Explicit Peer Review

To avoid the difficulties of the implicit approach, there has been increasing emphasis on the explicit format,[9,10] though Lembcke, as early as 1956, suggested the use of explicit criteria to ensure objectivity and reliability.[11]

This format outlines, for any given diagnostic entity or problem, a series of measures and procedures which peer consensus indicates could or should occur for the patient with the given condition. Charts are then reviewed, generally retrospectively, to see whether such criteria are met.

The disadvantage of such an approach is the temptation to create a "laundry" list of required items whose main effect may be to escalate the cost of care without clear indication that the quality has been similarly affected. There are also difficulties when concomitant disease exists and plays a major role in the patient's response, e.g., to assess care of diabetes as adequate in a patient who dies from untreated pyelonephritis, is an exercise in sophistry.

Another "potential difficulty with explicit process auditing is that the use of a limited number of health problems for which explicit criteria can be developed may sensitize providers to those problems, and thus, not accurately reflect the overall care provided."[12]

The advantage of this approach is that the problems of subjectivity and reproducibility are avoided, although not totally excluded (for example, assessment of adequate components of a history contains a considerable amount of subjectivity). In addition, this approach can be more readily adapted to large numbers of cases for once the initial criteria are developed, the audit can be performed by nonphysician personnel, thus reducing cost, and to an unknown extent, can serve as a screen for identification of problems that fail to meet criteria. The number that do meet criteria and still are not well handled, has not been studied in sufficiently rigorous detail.

3. Criteria Mapping[13]

A potentially useful method is being developed by the University of California at Los Angeles EMCRO. This method, called "Criteria Mapping," utilizes sequential judgements based on quantitative data to assess quality by chart review. This method, employing second, third, and fourth generations of criteria, individualizes patients and, therefore, does not penalize the physician for appropriate omissions. Further, because of the use of specific quantitative information readily identifiable in the chart, the use of this method allows abstraction by nonprofessional abstractors. Also, because the criteria follow the branching logic of decision making, the method can be applied to conditions or complaints as well as diagnosed and standardized diseases. It is expected that the measurement of process by this method will correlate better with outcomes because it better reflects the quality of clinical performance.

Neither criteria mapping nor explicit criteria derived by a consensus method can overcome the problems of the nonrecording of critical information. One of the disadvantages of criteria mapping is that considerably more physician input and expertise are needed to construct a set of criteria. Studies to determine the feasibility of criteria mapping relative to other methods, and studies to determine the relation of various measures of process to each other and in relation to outcome, should result in more reliable and more valid assessment of quality of clinical performance.

The Clinical Trial As Evaluation Methodology The term "clinical" trial is defined for the purpose of this statement as "A medical experiment carried out on human subjects." Thus, in the very broad sense of the definition, any human being who was the recipient of a medical intervention could be considered a clinical trial consisting of one subject receiving a single treatment; i.e., a case history. At the other extreme, there are the huge double-blind randomized clinical trials using many subjects and many interventions followed in time. At the present time, current application of clinical trials applies primarily to curative medicine or secondary preventive health activities; application to primary preventive activities is limited.

In assessing the utility of the "clinical" trial as an evaluation methodology, the pros and cons of many types of clinical trials will need to be covered. These are shown in Tables 3, 4, and 5 as answers to a series of questions on clinical trials.

Clinical Outcome Measures

1. Introduction

The outcome approach to evaluation has only recently been revived from the days of Codman,[14] the Boston surgeon, who between the years 1912 and 1914, evaluated every case admitted to his hospital by "classifying the *results* as favorable or unfavorable, and assigning responsibility for the latter to errors in diagnostic and technical ability, poor surgical judgement, inadequate care or equipment, the type of disease or the patient's refusal of treatment."[15]

In the intervening years, little emphasis was given to measurement of outcome in a formally designed sense. In part, this was due to the general medical profession's antagonism or lack of interest in any form of evaluation; and lack of sufficient medical knowledge to delineate the

116

natural history of many diseases and numerous grey areas in medical therapeutics where evidence for long-term efficacy is lacking. As interest in this approach reemerged in the 1960s, the words, "outcome," "intermediate outcome," "end result," "output," etc., were often used interchangeably and the lack of standard definitions and common interpretation of these terms, even now, contributes to confusion.

In Sanazaro and Williamson's [16] provisional classification based on reports by internists (1968), a distinction was made between *patient end results* and *process outcomes*. DeGeyndt,[17] in 1969, referred to *output* as "the result of the performance of an activity" while *outcome* was the "attainment of a state of health by the patient, taking health in its broadest definitional sense." Williamson [18] (1971) pointed out differences in terms of *diagnostic outcomes* (representing the data required to determine the need for care, specific therapy, and prognosis) and *therapeutic outcomes* (representing care in terms of health status). In 1974, Gonella and Zeleznik [19] stated that "every health care *outcome* should be evaluated in terms of its being the results of an interplay of at least four categories of factors which may be identified as follows: the performance of the physician; the adequacy of the technical setting in which the physician offers his services; the patient receiving the health care services; the social and physical environment in which the health care services are provided," a statement much in line with Codman's five areas for assigning responsibility, developed 63 years ago.

In addition to the approach's only recent reemergence and the semantic difficulties, there had developed, to a minor extent, a polarization between the outcome and process proponents. However, Donabedian [20] has stated that process and outcome are intimately related. Though he does not suggest that a combination word be actually used to show their interrelatedness, nevertheless, he points out with the words "outcess" and "procome," that they form one continuum in the care and cure sequence. Just as Hutchison [21] pointed out intervention points in a disease continuum, so Barro [22] quotes Simon as suggesting that "process and outcome should be viewed as a continuous chain of events composed of many links with each link representing an outcome. Each of these links is an intermediate outcome that can be evaluated." Williamson [23] recently stated that "the issue should not be outcome or process or structure, but rather when and where to apply each of these valid methods, utilizing their strengths to improve patient health."

2. Application (Pros and Cons)

Efforts to apply outcome measures utilize (1) retrospective chart audit, and (2) patient interviews as in Hagner's et al.[24] retrospective assessment of patient outcome in a comprehensive medicine clinic. A third method is by direct verification, for example, "misdiagnosis" and

Table 3. Characteristics of Clinical Trials

TYPE—CONTROLS	PURPOSE	ASSIGNMENT OF IVM[a] AND SELECTION OF CONTROLS	KNOWLEDGE OF IVM(S)	THIRD-PARTY EVALUATION
Single Case Trial (no controls)	Formulation of new hypotheses.	The single case is selected on judgment basis.	Known by both clinician and patient.	None
Nonrandomized Historical or Literature Controls	Estimation of IVM effect rather than comparison with a control.	No randomicity for trial people; probably some bias in the controls.	Known by clinician.	Sometimes, but not usually.
Controls from Previous Study	Estimate IVM effect; compare with previous study as controls.	No randomicity for trial people; control selection dependent on specific previous study.	Known by clinician and trial people.	Yes, it can be done this way.
"Matched" Ongoing Study	Comparison of IVM(s) with a control.	The IVM is assigned to the person in need. Then, one looks for similar person not in experiment as matched control and follows concurrently during trial.	Known by clinician and trial people.	Sometimes, it should be done this way.
Completely Randomized Placebo Control	Comparison of IVM with a placebo.	Trial people selected randomly; controls unknown to investigator.	The clinician is aware of the total experimental protocol, but does not know which IVM, placebo, etc., goes to which person. The patient is informed about the experiment and consents to be a part of the trial.	Always. There must be a peer review committee and an objective administrator, analyst on the trial.
Intervention Modality Control	Comparison of new IVM(s) with a standard IVM.	Trial people selected randomly; controls unknown to investigator.		
"Matched" Controls (blocking)	Comparison of IVM(s) with either a standard IVM or placebo.	Trial people selected randomly; controls unknown to investigator.		
Stratified Randomized Placebo Control	Comparison of an IVM(s) with a placebo in each stratum.	Within stratum, people are randomly assigned to IVM(s) and placebo.		

| Intervention Modality Control | Comparison of a new IVM(s) with a standard IVM in each stratum. | Within stratum, people are randomly assigned to IVM(s) |
| "Matched Controls (blocking) | Comparison of IVM with either a standard IVM or a placebo in each stratum. | Within stratum, patients are matched. IVM(s) are randomly assigned to matched people. |

a Intervention Modality.

Table 4. Characteristics of Clinical Trials

TYPE	DIFFICULTY OF ADMINISTERING	SAMPLE SIZE REQUIRED	COST
Single Case Trial (no controls)	None	One	Trivial
Nonrandomized Historical or Literature Controls	None	One-half as large as the random-ized trial for the same trial; can be done with small numbers.	Least expensive
Controls from previous study	None	One-half as large; can be done with small numbers.	Least expensive
"Matched" Ongoing Study	Most difficult of the non-randomized trials but easier . than all the randomized trials.	Ranks a distant second behind the randomized trial; can be done with few people with careful selection of the on-going controls.	A distant fifth
Completely Randomized Placebo Control and Intervention Modality Control	If large scale and cooperative, difficult to administer.	The size depends on the differ-ence expected between IVM and control. If the new IVM is a small modification or the mea-sure of success subjective, *large numbers are required*; if large difference, small numbers will do.	Fourth highest
"Matched" Controls (blocking)	Requires tight control, more than any above.	Good blocking will require fewer people than trials with completely randomized controls.	Second highest
Stratified Randomized Placebo Control and Intervention Modality Control	If large scale and cooperative one, difficult to administer.	The size of the trial depends on the difference expected be-tween IVM and control. If the	Third highest

| "Matched" Controls (blocking) | This is the most difficult to administer, since a little mix-up will invalidate a large study. | new IVM is a small modification or the measure of success subjective, large numbers are required; if large difference, small numbers will do. Good blocking will require fewer people than trials with completely randomized controls. | Most costly |

Table 5. Characteristics of Clinical Trials

TYPE	ETHICAL PROBLEMS	VALID STATISTICAL INFERENCE	WARNINGS TO BE EMPHASIZED
Single Case Trial	None	None, but many new potentially successful intervention modalities arise this way, e.g., smallpox inoculations.	All that can be said is that it is a sample size n = 1. It can lead to hypotheses for testing in a more scientific manner.
Nonrandomized Historical or Literature Controls		Comparative statistics and, to a large extent, statistical inference are hazardous.	Use of historical controls is suspect. If one insists on doing this kind of trial, the choice of historical controls should be made by an outside peer.
Controls from previous study	The argument goes that the intervention modality being used is the best known (according to the physician/program). Thus, ethically it is the only way to do the trial.	If the previous study controls were from a randomized trial, assumptions needed for acceptable statistical inferences are not too difficult to handle.	Yes. Previous study controls are better than historical controls, but not the best type with which to compare an IVM. Great care needs to be taken to insure no biased interpretation. Controls should be selected by third party.
"Matched" (ongoing) Study		Yes, if the matched controls are well selected in a fashion that meets rather severe statistical requirements.	The major problem is lack of a true control. The ongoing matched control is as close to a placebo as one can get. The choice of these controls must be done independently of the experimenter by a third party. The clinician should never know what is happening in the matched control.

122

All completely
randomized and
stratified
randomized trials

A matter of opinion. Complete understanding of both the individual and program/doctor is needed. A peer review committee and good analytical procedures minimize the ethical concerns in some instances.

Of all the kinds of trials, the statistical validity of these kinds of randomized trials is superior.

Although a double-blind randomized trial has been conducted, the final analysis should carefully check to make sure the IVM and control groups are reasonably balanced with respect to known demographic, etc., ie., factors that might bias the conclusions.

"missed" heart failures, i.e., measurement of the staff's diagnostic effectiveness in Williamson's[25] sampling of heart failure suspects in the Baltimore City Hospital Emergency Room. For a limited number of conditions, however, outcome studies can be effective and of great value. The classic studies of hypertensive patients by the Veterans Administration,[26] and response of childhood anemia to therapy,[27] are two.

In many instances, the application of outcome measurements poses particular problems. Sanazaro and Williamson[16] state that "it is recognized that only a minor proportion of the physician's professional efforts (or a preventive health program's efforts) involve the application of technical, chemical, biological or physical modalities . . . at present, there is no practical technique for analyzing the 'other actions' of physicians (or programs) which do not involve scientifically validated principles and modalities." Little work has been carried out on defining sufficiently the variables of patient behavior,[28] physician behavior,[29] and program environment which contribute to and affect the patient's response to care and reflect intermediate outcomes in provider performance levels and patient compliance.

Another problem in the application of outcome measures consists of the fact that "the natural history of illness and possible benefits of medical intervention are not known with enough precision to permit valid outcome measures to be established. . . . Often, intermediate clinical outcomes are not available or are medically controversial. Control of blood sugar in diabetics is a case in point. If maintenance of a normal blood sugar were associated with a decrease in diabetic complications, the blood sugar level could be utilized as an intermediate outcome. The possible association is medically controversial and, therefore, a blood sugar is of debatable validity as an intermediate outcome measurement."[12]

Williamson[23] also considers this a major disadvantage of outcome assessment, i.e., "the fact that research data are often unavailable for establishing causal relations between medical care process and patient health outcomes. The dearth of adequate data regarding the sensitivity and specificity of diagnostic methods or the efficacy of therapeutic interventions can seriously limit the outcome approach unless alternative means are applied to manage these information deficits. Although this data deficit handicaps all approaches to quality assessment, it is especially noticeable with outcome methods in which standards depend considerably on consensus regarding assumptions of causality."

Morehead[5] has stated that "such studies of this nature are time consuming, require careful study design and . . . what is needed, as both the public and financers of medical services become increasingly concerned about the quality of the product delivered, is a relatively simple tool that can be applied in a variety of settings, is relatively inexpensive,

124

and will act as a screen to identify an area of major concern: unacceptable technical performance by the health care provider."

The Tracer Approach As formulated by Kessner and associates[30-34] under the auspices of the Institute of Medicine, National Academy of Sciences, the "tracer method" of evaluating health services for ambulatory patients is not, in fact, a single method. Rather, it constitutes a strategy or framework for evaluation that utilizes a number of specific evaluation foci, research methods, and data sources to accomplish its purpose.

1. Scope of Concern

At the core of the strategy is the dual premise that carefully selected health problems or morbidity conditions may serve as indicators of the health status of a defined population, and as focal points ("tracers") for the evaluation of health care delivery within the defined population.

The strategy includes evaluation of the outcome of care, the clinical process of care, and the structure of care (provider qualifications and organizational setting). Equally important, it entails design, analysis, and interpretation of such evaluative efforts in the light of patient and population characteristics.

Health care evaluation strategies containing some or all of these elements have been advanced by others.[18,35-43] What is distinctive about the tracer strategy, therefore, is not its scope but its utilization of specific conditions to link key elements in the evaluation framework.

2. Selection of Tracers

In order to be eligible for use as a tracer, a health condition must meet certain criteria.[32] Specifically, the condition must be functionally significant for those affected, easy to diagnose, relatively prevalent in the population, and responsive to medical care intervention. In addition, the techniques of medical management for the condition should be well defined for at least one of the following processes: prevention, diagnosis, treatment, and rehabilitation or adjustment. Finally, the epidemiology of the condition should be well understood so that the effects of socioeconomic factors on the prevalence of the condition can be taken into account.

A single tracer need not furnish the basis for evaluation of every aspect of health care. It must, however, illuminate at least one aspect, e.g., prevention, screening, evaluation, management, or follow-up of health problems. A basic assumption of the strategy is that a properly selected *set* of tracers will permit evaluation of all aspects of health care.[32,33]

3. Application of Tracer Strategy: Some Requirements

Application of the tracer strategy requires a defined population whose demographic characteristics are known, in order that appropriate tracer conditions may be selected. It also requires formulation of explicit criteria against which services delivered can be compared, including definitions of satisfactory and unsatisfactory outcomes of care.

In the only field trial of the tracer approach undertaken thus far,[33] additional methodological desiderata are evident, as the following over-simplified summary indicates.

4. Field Trial of Strategy

Having selected and justified middle-ear infection and associated hearing loss, iron-deficiency anemia, and vision defects as tracers to be used in the evaluation of children's medical care and health status in Washington, D.C., Kessner and associates[33] first carried out a sample interview survey of households in two socioeconomically different communities, chosen on the basis of census data. Through the survey they identified nearly 2,800 children's usual source of care, their tracer-specific medical histories, and their family's socioeconomic characteristics and medical experience. Through interviews they also obtained the same information about an additional sample of 672 children whose families were enrolled at a neighborhood health center located outside of the two communities.

The investigators then determined the children's health status (outcome of care) with respect to the tracer conditions through direct clinical examination of the children by physicians using protocols in a special clinic, to which children were transported after appropriate permissions had been secured.

The process of care was evaluated for the tracer conditions, using explicit criteria, on the basis of abstracts of charts of a sample of the children examined, supplemented with information provided by questionnaires sent to the physicians named as the children's usual source of care.

The physician questionnaires also provided information about the structure of care: the organizational setting of the physicians' practice, the physicians' medical training, and their attitudes and satisfactions. This information was supplemented by demographic data concerning the physicians obtained from the American Medical Association.

It is not yet clear whether all of these research procedures and data sources used in the field trial constitute equally necessary methodological components of the tracer strategy. Conceivably some could be dispensed with or simplified, as occurs in the hypothetical example of application of the strategy to evaluation of a neighborhood health center advanced by Kessner et al.[30,32,34] and in his study of infant mortality.[31]

It is clear, however, that the field trial uncovered a pattern of rather poor care as indicated by both process and outcome data, and that differences within this pattern seemed to be associated more with variations in the socioeconomic status and education of the children's parents than with variations in the characteristics and organization of the physicians providing care.

5. Usefulness for Evaluating Preventive Health Care

As a strategy for evaluating the quality of health care delivery, the tracer approach is elegant in conception though unwieldy in application.

Strongly in its favor are its comprehensive scope of concern and its abstemious use of a limited number of specific health problems as focal points for examining and linking more general elements in the evaluation framework. In the words of the originators of the strategy:

> The frequency rates of tracer conditions gauge the health status of a population; the ratio of treated to untreated cases measures the proficiency of the delivery system in reaching its community; the processes of diagnosis and treatment, when compared to a set of criteria, reflect the quality of medical practice; and the outcome of the treatment highlights the composite social and medical environment to which the patient is exposed.[32]

Further, the strategy is flexible in that, within certain limits, it apparently may be tailored to examine either primary or secondary preventive health care, or both.

As a strategy for determining general health status of a given population, however, the tracer approach appears less promising. Given the tracer conditions selected thus far (middle-ear infection and associated hearing loss; visual disorders; iron-deficiency anemia; essential hypertension; urinary tract infections; cervical cancer,[32] generalization from tracer-specific health status to general health status seems hazardous at best.

Conceptual issues aside, a major disadvantage of the tracer strategy is the extensive and methodologically complex data base required for its implementation. As presently outlined, such a data base would appear to be too costly and cumbersome to maintain and utilize for routine, periodic monitoring of health care delivery systems.

Another problem stems from the stringent criteria that must be met in order for a health condition to qualify as a tracer. These criteria effectively screen out from scrutiny a variety of health conditions that might nevertheless be of considerable interest on other grounds. This is to suggest that, in cases where the health program objective is limited to prevention, screening, or treatment of a particular disease that does not meet tracer criteria, application of the tracer strategy to evaluate the program would be inappropriate.

6. Further Research

Additional strengths and weaknesses of the tracer strategy may come to light as further research using the strategy is undertaken.

The originators of the approach quite reasonably suggest that such research should include testing the methodology in a variety of health service programs, and expansion of the number and type of tracer sets to facilitate better representation of age groups, types of disorders, and kinds of services.[32] Further research should also include experimentation with less time-consuming and less costly sources and methods of data collection. Desirable in addition would be empirical examination of how—and whether—a meaningful index of general health status might be formed from an expanded set of tracer conditions. Finally, it would be useful to explore the extent to which the tracer approach to ambulatory care evaluation can be articulated with current systems and methods of evaluating inpatient hospital care.

Other Methodologies

1. Critical Incident Technique

"The occurrence of any major adverse event which is significantly preventable, given present technology, represents a possible failure which requires investigation, so that one may determine who or what must carry responsibility for its occurrence. This procedure uses each adverse event to burrow backwards into the web of prior care, seeking weaknesses subject to remedy. It is perhaps not overly fanciful to suggest that, if a sufficiently broad range of adverse outcomes is identified, to include psychological and social states as well as physical or physiological, one would have a 'retroactive tracer' strategy of evaluation as a complement to the prospective 'tracer methodology' formulated by Kessner."[20]

2. Staging (Secondary Prevention)

The basic premise of the "staging" concept is that the seriousness of a patient's condition at some point in the treatment process is an indication of the outcome of the previous treatment. The general hypothesis for applying staging to quality assessment is that if a given population is not adequately handled by the medical care system ... then it can be expected, on the average, the population will tend to be farther advanced in illness than a population that is adequately cared for.

Disease staging involves defining different levels of severity for specific medical problems. The method calls for separating a medical problem or disease into three stages: Stage 1, Disease with no complications or problem of minimal severity; Stage II, Disease with local complications or problem of moderate severity; Stage III, Disease with systematic complications or problem of a serious nature.[44]

Laboratory Modalities

The health laboratory is an essential tool in both primary and secondary preventive health programs. The degree to which this tool is effective depends upon a number of factors, among which are "state of the art" relevance of laboratory tests for the particular preventive problem, the quality of test performance (accuracy and precision) available, and the comparability of test results from laboratory to laboratory and from time to time.

Laboratory tests may be used to choose those individuals in a population who are to receive primary preventive care (immunization) or be subjected to dietary control (phenylketonuria), as well as a means of preclinical case finding. The relevance of the laboratory test and its screening effectiveness (false negative/false positive) are determined by basic physiopathological factors, but they are also greatly affected by the "sharpness" of the laboratory tool (method) employed. The relationships of these factors are outlined in two of many recent papers [45,46] that could be cited and in two books published by the World Health Organization. [47,48]

The effectiveness of laboratory tools in preventive medicine (when they can be used) rests upon:

1. an inherent difference detectable between subsets of population groups;
2. an inherent capability of a laboratory test to detect this difference (or some parameter related to this difference); and
3. the reliability of the laboratory test as it is actually used to detect subset differences.

Obviously, these parts of the problem interact. An unreliable test may obscure a very significant inherent difference between population subsets. Poorly defined population subsets (children versus adult; male versus female; fasting versus nonfasting; immune versus nonimmune) may obscure the results of a reliable laboratory test. However, assuming the existence of a significant relevant subset difference, the reliability of the laboratory test applied to the preventive disease problem is critical.

The test itself is used to define the laboratory limits of normality in a population subset determined to be normal on other grounds. After the limits of normality have been established for the laboratory test, the test can be applied to the population at risk, and decision points may be set so as to achieve an appropriate sensitivity/specificity ratio for the particular disease being studied.

The sensitivity/specificity ratio is critically affected by the two quality components of laboratory test performance—precision and accuracy. The precision of the test (i.e., the ability to get the same result repeatedly) obviously will affect the screening capability of any single application of the test. The accuracy of the test (the ability to get the "correct" result) has the same effect, although it is not so obvious. The effect of the test's inaccuracy on screening effectiveness is related directly to the initial process by which the normal or "screening range" is established. If the screening range is established by an accurate (zero-bias) procedure and the population is actually screened by an inaccurate procedure (i.e., having significant bias), the sensitivity/specificity ratio is markedly altered.

An example of the problems raised by inaccurate testing was reported in November 1974, in a "Preliminary Report on Cost-Effectiveness of Urine Testing," prepared for the National Institute on Drug Abuse, Department of Health, Education, and Welfare."[49] The study was concerned with defining the total costs of urine testing for methadone maintenance programs, and in addition examined the problems surrounding laboratory proficiency. The conclusion concerning the latter was that: "urine testing results are so inaccurate as to preclude any attempt to determine if they are really of any use. . . ." For example, "the Department of Defense blind proficiency testing results, covering nearly a million tests done between November 1971 and January 1972 (by three commercial laboratories) showed that these laboratories identified correctly only 50 to 65 percent of the quality control samples submitted." One of the resulting recommendations following numerous similar examples was: "CDC needs, via legislation, more power to severely restrict or eliminate the activities of laboratories that do not meet the stringent standards which need to be set up. The results of not taking action in this regard could be disastrous for clients and for treatment programs. If laboratories cannot be regulated strictly through licensure, training, education, etc., and if the level of proficiency cannot be improved, elimination of urine testing (in such programs) should be considered. . . ."

As the above points out, there are marked tendencies of laboratories, even under the best of circumstances, to exhibit individual laboratory bias (or inaccuracy) which affects screening effectiveness locally and also the epidemiological interpretation when data are collected from many different laboratories.

Evaluation of the reliability of single laboratories, with respect to accuracy and precision, rests upon the availability of reference methods and materials characterized by such methods. Reference methods and materials have been available for common diagnostically useful constituents, in general only from commercial sources, each company making its own decisions and control guides. This has produced almost a state of chaos, especially in areas in which the technological constraints of instrumentation have been a factor.

130

In 1967 the Federal Government assumed an active role in assuring quality performance in clinical laboratories. More recently, the Food and Drug Administration (FDA) has been developing standards for the performance of products intended for use in clinical and other health laboratories. Center for Disease Control and the National Bureau of Standards (NBS) serve as prime technical advisors to the FDA in this field, which will lead to the development of national reference methods and reference materials. These federal efforts should bring about an increase in the precision and accuracy of clinical laboratory measurement.

Nonfederal efforts to promote the quality of laboratory performance should not go unnoticed. They antedated the more recent federal activity and if uniformly strengthened, should form the basis for local and regional efforts at laboratory quality controls. Over the years, the College of American Pathologists, the American Association of Bioanalysts, the privately operated Proficiency Testing Service (Dr. William Sunderman), many states, and other regional groups have undertaken interlaboratory comparisons (essentially relative accuracy tests).

For example, in New York State, external quality control is carried out by the State Laboratory in Albany. Unknowns are sent which are performed by the tested laboratories and the results are sent back to the central examining agency and compared to reference laboratories as well as to the other peer laboratories. The most highly specialized and staffed laboratories in the region are often designated as reference laboratories. In addition, examiners or inspectors at various levels of laboratory expertise may be sent to visit the laboratories and make appropriate on-site visits. However, it must be emphasized that any such system of surveillance must have a self-examination system built in. There is a tendency to regard the examining agency and the reference laboratories as automatically correct and gospel. But there are still many flaws and loopholes in such control systems and a very strict self-questioning attitude must prevail.

In any program of country-wide increase in laboratory testing, regional laboratory development would be appropriate. These laboratories would then be the reference laboratories for the surrounding area as well as the central laboratories for the specialized and difficult tests. These laboratories would permit the necessary effective operation and sophistication of equipment to extend an umbrella of supervision over smaller adjoining laboratories. A system of quality control of these larger central laboratories could be easily organized on a state- or country-wide basis.

This system of control using the reference laboratories and a central agency may be applied to the commercial laboratories in similar fashion. The largest commercial laboratories have established solid reputations and many are used by teaching hospitals and academic institutions. The small commercial operations, however, lend themselves to many shortcuts and attempts by single technicians to cover all or many areas of laboratory procedures. Then laboratories must be subject to careful review and control with limitation in areas of activity.

It is particularly difficult to monitor the laboratory work done in the individual physician's office. But he should be restricted to performance of relatively simple laboratory procedures on his own patients. Again, the regional (reference) laboratories could help control and survey these laboratories and also take into account the many local variations that obtain in different parts of the country.

Surveillance of the utilization (over and under) of laboratory procedures and billing practices are problems of different magnitude and complexity and require entirely different approaches. In the area of billing, it is recommended that the patient be billed directly for any laboratory work done. Any system which places the physician in any way between the laboratory and the patient encourages many forms of collusion between physician and laboratory to the possible detriment of the patient.

Effective use of the laboratory in preventive health care requires that it provide accurate and precise results. Efforts to assure such results include establishing local and regional quality control centers; federal licensing and certification of laboratories; and private, state and federal surveillance of actual laboratory performance. Technical improvements and adoption and use of common reference materials and methods are integral essential parts of the total process.

Health Education Modalities: Methods Available to Evaluate the Health Education Components of Preventive Health Programs:

Definition and Inclusions

The health education components of preventive health programs may be considered to include:

1. Communications directed at the public and at patients and families to influence knowledge, attitudes, beliefs and norms supporting health practices.

2. Community organization activities designed to influence the voluntary adjustment of resources to make health services more accessible and acceptable to the populations in need of these services.

3. Staff development activities, such as consultation, supervision, in-service training and continuing education designed to influence the attitudes and behavior of providers towards patients and clients so as to reinforce appropriate health behavior in the public.[50]

The common feature of these three modalities of health education, and therefore, the defining characteristics of health education strategies, is that they are designed to bring about voluntary changes in health-related behavior. This distinguishes educational strategies from legal, administrative, environmental control, political, medical, and other strategies, although health education may be used in support of these alternative strategies.

Outcomes Measured in the Evaluation of Health Education

The immediate outcomes of the three health education modalities are identified in Fig. 1 as (1) *predisposing* factors, (2) *enabling* factors, and (3) *reinforcing* factors. These factors are viewed as antecedent to behavioral changes which are sought in preventive health programs. Indicators and dimensions of behavioral measurement for the evaluation of health education outcomes are listed below "Behavioral Problems" in Fig. 1. Measures of the more immediate (antecedent) variables to the left provide "process" evaluation in health education.[50]

Input Measurement in Evaluation of Health Education

Because behavioral changes are dependent on a variety of antecedent variables (predisposing, enabling, and reinforcing factors), each of which must be influenced by a distinct educational input, the evaluation of health education programs or strategies must be distinguished from evaluation of specific health education techniques or tactics. The latter may be related on a theoretical level with the specific outcomes each is expected to influence, as in Table 6, but the outcomes are maximized in practice by the combination of various inputs.[50] These and related considerations in the design of health education programs have implications for the appropriate adaptation and analysis of experimental and quasi-experimental designs to evaluate health education.[51-52] The measurement of inputs must similarly take into account factors specific to the educational process and educational technology, such as the usual relationship between unit costs and effectiveness,[53] economies of scale in informational technologies,[54] the logarithmic diffusion curve in the penetration of community programs,[50,55] the quality of educational media,[56-57] personnel used,[55,58-63] and the setting and circumstances of the educational encounter or exposure.[64]

The methods and instruments to measure these input variables have been variously developed but are far from standardized except where simple counts are possible, as in the number of pamphlets distributed, number of home visits made, hours of mass media time used, etc.[65]

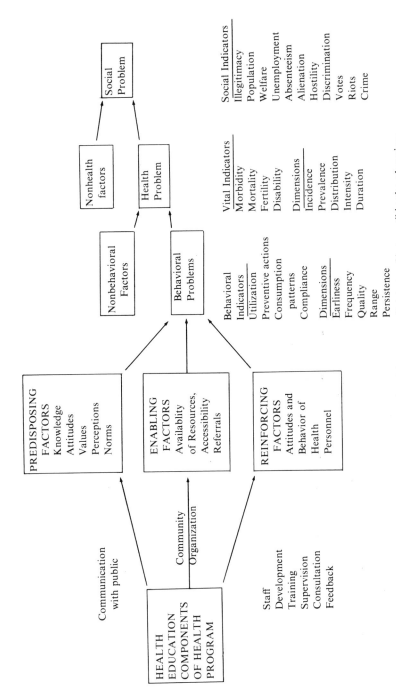

Figure 1. Approximate relationships among "objects of interest" in the planning and evaluation of health education.

Table 6. Theoretical relationships between some specific educational components of a health program and the expected benefits.

EDUCATIONAL INPUT (Cost)	BEHAVIORAL OUTCOME	MEDICAL OR ADMINISTRATIVE BENEFIT
Showing concern and interest for needs of the patient or population	Patient satisfaction	Public support for the program or agency Payment of bills by patients Reduced malpractice suits Kept appointments (Reduced broken appointments) Competitive with quacks and other alternatives
Communication of information	Patient knowledge, attitudes, beliefs	Compliance Better diagnosis
Entertainment or other appeal to motives and values of the patient	Patient interest Reduced boredom	Reduced delay Kept appointments
Communication with relatives	Social support for patient	Compliance; public support
Outreach	Public awareness, interest, attitudes, preventive health behavior	Patient recruitment Primary prevention Appropriate utilization
In-Service training	Staff awareness, interest, attitudes, showing concern	Patient satisfaction Patient knowledge (see above)
Community organization	Coordination of resources, referrals, social support for patients	Appropriate utilization Patient recruitment Reduced duplication Public support
Mass communication	Public awareness, interest, some social support, some knowledge	Public support Patient recruitment Reduced delay
Follow-up contact with former patients	Patient reinforcement, sustained interest and commitment	Return appointments Continued adoption (persistence, compliance)

Measuring Prebehavioral Outcomes of Health Education

There are widely standardized measurement instruments available for some health-related knowledge inventories and attitude scales. Unfortunately, the better standardized tools tend to measure the least important health beliefs and attitudes. The most documented set of health beliefs known to be related to a variety of health behaviors, for example, is almost totally without standardization, tests of reliability or of validity.[66] Knowledge inventories and attitude scales are relatively well standardized, on the other hand, in trivial areas by health behavior criteria.[67] Personality measures are the most extensively and thoroughly tested and standardized scales,[68] but fail repeatedly to explain more than a tenth of the variance in most health behaviors, with the notable exception of the internal-external "Locus of Control" scale,[69] and possibly the "Value Orientation" scale.[70] Measures of predisposing demographic variables are better standardized than psychological variables, with most of the standardization following U.S. Census Bureau procedures, but some being adapted to reflect social psychological predispositions or to maximize the variance accounted for in health behavior.[71-75] Measures of relative exposure and reactions to various mass media, such as the Nielsen ratings, are well developed.[76-80]

Community organization outcomes are the most difficult to evaluate in most health education programs because of the difficulty of controlling extraneous factors influencing the outcomes. Case studies have been the major source of evaluative information,[81] particularly in the analysis of interorganizational relationships.[82] Considerable efforts in recent years have yielded new methods and procedures for measuring process and outcomes of consumer participation in health planning.[83-85] Another influence of community organization on enabling factors that has received increased methodological development is health referral patterns.[86]

Staff development outcomes are now receiving increased attention with the growing interest in continuing education and new manpower configurations in health services. Evaluation of training programs and of supervision has traditionally been limited to "reactionaries" asking trainees or supervisors how they liked various aspects of their supervisor or the training program.[87,88] The gradual adoption of more formal use of task analysis and instructional objectives by trainers has given impetus and greater feasibility to the evaluation of behavioral outcomes in training and supervision.[89-91] These developments have also improved the prospects for evaluation of consultation,[92] and of institutional and continuing education.[93-96]

From the standpoint of health education in preventive health programs, the process to which these staff development activities are addressed is improved attitudes and behavior of staff toward patients. Instruments focused specifically on these process variables are emerging in a variety of contexts.[63,94,95,97-101]

Measuring Behavioral Outcomes of Health Education.

Standardized measures of behavioral outcomes are better developed than measures of the antecedent and process variables discussed above, but agreement on methods and procedures for collecting, analyzing, and interpreting behavioral measures is far from unanimous. The most extensive methodological work has been with indices of health service utilization.[102] Recent reviews of the literature, however, reveal wide discrepancies on criteria of "adequate" or "appropriate" utilization in terms of delay,[103,104] and the frequency or duration of return appointments.[105-111]

Greater discrepancies are found in the measurement of preventive health practices,[71,73,112-114] in compliance with medical regimens,[114-117] and in risk-reduction behavior (screening tests, smoking, weight control, diet, etc.).[55,112,116,118] The overlap among these behavioral categories is part of the problem but the lack of agreement on measures of behavior within categories is not eliminated by reclassification.

Study Design and Evaluation of Three Levels Involved in Persuasion Formulated by Cartwright.

The "Three Town Heart Disease Prevention Program"[119] attempted to measure (1) changes in people's cognitive structure—in their level of information, (2) changes in motivational structure—in what they want to do (attitude), and (3) changes in their action structure—in what they do (behavior).

The study objective was to learn cost effective and human effective means of helping people to reduce risk. "We needed to know how far short, if any, . . . a mass media communication effect alone would fall from a more ideal one in which personal instruction employing behavior modification and other methods would supplement the mass media campaign.

The study design was as follows:

> We sought towns which were more or less self-contained communities with their own mass media systems . . . as well as like one another as possible in important demographic characteristics . . . It was especially important that the control community be outside the mass media orbit of the other two towns.

The initial survey consisted of household interviews to determine the information base on diet, exercise, and smoking, plus physical examinations. "Over 80 percent of the drawn samples were both interviewed and examined."

The next stage included a mass media campaign in towns W and G utilizing television, radio, newspapers (doctors' columns and dietary columns), print items such as booklets, cookbooks, etc., which were mailed to residents, and business cards and billboards. In addition, in town W, an intensive instruction program on diet, exercise, and smoking was implemented on a subsample of high-risk subjects. The behavior modification strategy developed was based on the theoretical work of Albert Bandura which contains a five-part process: (1) Analysis of existing relevant behavior and behavioral objectives, (2) modeling of new

137

acts by instructor or model, (3) guided practice of new behavior by the learner, (4) reinforcement of the new behavior, and (5) maintenance of the new behavior without further instructor intervention.

Reinforcement devices for various new behaviors of all three sorts—diet, smoking, and exercise—included instructor and spouse encouragement, group support, weekly weigh-ins, the progress report feedback system, and the anticipated gratification from doing well in the physical examinations to come.

The third town, T, served as a control town and received neither the mass media campaign nor the intensive instruction.

The evaluation of the program utilized three (reported) methods to determine change: (1) Interviews to determine attitude change, (2) medical data change, and (3) observation of community changes, e.g., "substantial drops in egg consumption took place in the entire sample of all three communities, with significant gains from W of greater magnitude than for G, but G showed comparably more gain than did the control community of Tracy."

Conclusions

"It is by no means evident as yet that the Cornfield risk reductions took place via changes in information, attitudes, and behavior. We are very much in the process of further analyses of these results.

The changes that took place via intensive instruction are clearly superior to those via mass media only. However, it is also clear that mass media only when applied to the learning of appropriate skills can be effective too. What we need now is to learn how to apply the maximum treatment via cost and human effective means. With the development and use of mass media in which skills learning is appropriately emphasized, it should be possible to make considerably greater gains in risk reduction behavior than we have thus far achieved. Recently we have experimented with a full-hour television program in which we ask viewers to score themselves on risk. In the process, they practice what is being shown and are fed back the correct responses. Previous film learning experiments (Michael and Maccoby) have shown this to be a highly effective instructional method. The stability of risk reduction behavior change is of course of great concern, and we are continuing to study our three communities to determine how durable the newly acquired habits are."

Implications for Future Evaluation of Health Education.

The major obstacle to advancing the scientific base of health education practice in preventive health programs is clearly the paucity of

138

standardized measures of both input and outcome variables. This precludes the comparison of findings between studies and limits the generalizability of results. The scientific and professional literature related to health education is mushrooming in both the behavioral science and the health science journals, but it lacks the cumulative quality essential to the codification of knowledge and the development of theory and policy.

Program Results

1. Reduction of Incidence and Health Status: Preventive program results are measured primarily in terms of morbidities and mortalities prevented, at the primary or secondary levels, as a demonstrable result of the program. These are the central and obvious outcomes to be measured, but care must be taken that "program results" are truly results of the program, rather than of other intervening variables occurring at the same time.

With the changing character of public health problems and increasing expectations of the public as to effectiveness of health care, morbidity and mortality data alone are but the first level of screening for program effectiveness. There has been increasing interest in defining and classifying varying degrees of health status of a population in order to measure functional status as an index of effectiveness of programs directed toward "slowing the progress of disease and conserving maximal function." (Definition of the American College of Preventive Medicine.) Behavioral modification leading to improved health habits, as well as compliance with therapeutic regimens, should be also examined in relation to programs both with specific and more generalized preventive health objectives.

2. Other Program Results: As difficult as such outcomes can be to measure and evaluate, there are yet other results which may be significant and even more difficult to measure. Other positive results are diverse and include, for example, reassurance to individuals resulting from negative results of a screening test, creation of new jobs, and the priming of local economy as a result of infusion of funds for the preventive program itself; and, on the minus side, use of funds for the program resulting in the funds not being used for another possibly more beneficial health or social program. These kinds of results tend to merge with "benefits," in the broad sense, becoming very value-laden, and are, therefore, usually conveniently neglected.

Reduction of Incidence.

Disease prevention has been effectively measured in the past primarily in the field of infectious disease by examination of legally mandated morbidity and mortality statistics. For specific diseases and conditions, field trials have established effectiveness (e.g., polio, fluoridation for dental caries) or noneffectiveness (e.g., influenza, viral upper respiratory disease), and have led to acceptance, limited acceptance, or rejection of the various intervention modalities as primary preventive health tools.

In the field of chronic disease, evidence is more difficult to accumulate, requires longer periods of time, and is complicated by the presence of intervening variables (cholesterol, obesity, exercise in heart disease).

The effects of early detection of disease on mortality and morbidity are beginning to show mixed patterns. There is general acceptance of early therapy in hypertension [26] but questions are beginning to be raised about the effectiveness of early detection of cancer of the cervix, [120,121] lung cancer, or breast cancer in younger age groups [122] in reducing mortality.

Therapeutic interventions to prevent morbidity and mortality are increasing as technical surgical skills increase (valve replacement, carotid endarterectomies; surgical intervention for CVAs, kidney transplants). Evaluations of such interventions are limited by small numbers of cases performed in isolated settings. However, increasing public awareness of such procedures will lead to demand so that it is imperative that data to evaluate effectiveness on a nationwide scale be undertaken. The randomized study of radical versus simple mastectomy for breast cancer [123] being mounted across the country is a good example of a concerted effort.

Health Status Evaluation.

The methodology in this field has evolved over a long period of time, mainly as a response to social forces. Nowhere is this more evident than in the efforts to develop methods to assess the status of the chronically ill. As early as the 1920s, state and local governments, recognizing the need to devise plans for the prevention, treatment, and care of chronic illness, conducted studies on the prevalence of these conditions. In the 1930s and 1940s, as the social and economic consequences of chronic disease became increasingly evident, other studies were conducted and the ordered classification of disability was introduced. During this same period, awareness increased of the need to develop new methods of solving the problems of chronic disease and serving the chronically ill; and in 1949, the Commission on Chronic Illness was established to work toward these ends. Their efforts produced many methodological contributions, among which were new insights into the classification of illness status.

In the years since, other researchers have continued the search for improved indices in order to plan and prescribe as they work toward beneficial outcomes. The purpose of these notes, then, is to examine some current approaches to the classification of the disability components of long-term illness status and to discuss the advantages and disadvantages of particular methods.

One approach to the classification of long-term disability is based on the concept of limitations of activity. As used by the National Center for Health Statistics in the United States National Health Survey, the chronically ill are classified according to the extent to which they are limited in their ability to carry on the major activity or social role considered appropriate for their age and/or sex group.[124] The concept also has been used by the Commission on Chronic Illness[125] and by the Social Security Administration[126] in their studies of the working-age population. It has the advantage of describing relatively objectively the role limitations imposed by chronic conditions and of delineating some of the rehabilitative and care needs of the chronically disabled. Classification based on this concept, however, does not deal with the functions or activities an individual should be able to perform in order to fulfill his normatively defined role.[127]

Classification systems based on the characterization of ill persons according to levels of functional capacity in walking, moving about the community, and performing self-care activities do attempt to assess these abilities. The Maryland Disability Index, also known as the Barthel Index, assesses movements and activities of daily living.[128] The Rapid Disability Rating Scale developed by Linn assesses, in addition, impairments in speech, hearing, sight, and mental status.[129] Katz's Index of ADL groups patients according to seven grades of dependence in bathing, dressing, going to toilet, transferring, continence, and feeding.[130,131] All of these systems provide measures of disability which are applicable to varied individual situations. In fact, mobility and self-care activities are perhaps a more realistic measure for the aged who have no major activity as such and who represent a large percentage of the chronically ill.

Classification systems based on this concept, however, do not fully explicate the varying patterns of disability which may occur among individuals with similar diagnoses, i.e., ". . . not all persons with the same pathological condition are disabled by it and, conversely, some persons appear to be disabled without detectable pathological conditions."[125] Thus, certain systems have been developed that combine criteria of disease and categories of function. The earliest attempt to develop such a dual system was made by the Baltimore Eastern Health District study which coded chronic diseases into six activity levels.[132] A decade later, the Commission on Chronic Illness developed a dual classification system in which individuals were divided into three groups: those with maximum disability regardless of diagnosis; those with less disability and some disease; and those with extended disability and no or minor disease.[133] Soon after, the Canadian Sickness Survey developed a scheme in which individuals "permanently" incapacitated by chronic conditions were classified into four activity levels.[134] All of these describe the activity losses which chronic conditions impose on affected persons.

Building on past knowledge, researchers recently have begun to adopt a profiled approach to classification in order to describe the outcome of disease in terms of disability and the likelihood of a poor outcome in the presence of associated major chronic disease. Katz et al. and James[135-138] have developed a method by which they classify chronically ill patients according to: (1) diagnosis based on categorical systems of chronic disease classification; (2) chronic disease abnormalities (or risk factors) identified through screening; and (3) scales of disability.

Within the National Center for Health Statistics, a clearinghouse on Health Indexes was created to provide a channel for information (e.g., a quarterly "Bibliography on Health Indexes") on the developing composite health status measures which reflect the positive side of health as well as morbidity and mortality.[139,140]

In summary, this review has not attempted to resolve problems, but to define them in ways that will perhaps contribute to the further development of improved methods of classification. Health practitioners and health managers require such systems in order to evaluate the effect of care on patients, place them in appropriate care facilities, monitor ongoing processes of care and allocate resources within programs serving the chronically ill.

Summary

The health care system of the United States is, consciously and otherwise, making choices at every level—from the federal to state to local to individual institutions and practitioners. The choices that are made in providing care are usually made in an immediate sense without taking into account a holistic view of the needs of the population being served and the opportunities for doing so through a range of elements of activity. This range covers the spectrum from primary prevention through secondary prevention, diagnosis, treatment, the control of disability, care without any hope of cure, and humanistic attention in terminal care.

It is of the utmost importance that evaluation and quality control be built into all preventive efforts so that their value may be objectively and precisely measured, thus providing a basis for comparison in setting priorities for health programs at every level and for providing feedback to delivery systems for improvement of services. Without such efforts, decisions about prevention treatment, cure, and care can only be made on a philosophic basis, clearly inadequate to serve the purposes of policy making in the health care field—at every level.

A public commitment by DHEW supported by policies, funding, and staff is necessary to achieve these objectives.

In formulation of an evaluation framework that could and should be applied to all programs, the Task Force developed a matrix (Table 1) for evaluation based on examining the components and objectives of a given program. This matrix enumerated five major areas that should be examined in the evaluation of any program or program element: (1) the proportion of population served (penetration rate); (2) cost efficiency; (3) structure and organization; (4) the process elements of provider input, support services, and health education; and (5) program results.

Whether it be a primary or secondary preventive health activity, any such program or program component should have clearly stated objectives, a defined delivery structure and organization, and standards for the modalities for implementation, be they clinical, supportive such as laboratory, x-ray, or pharmacy services, or in the field of health education.

The evaluation matrix was then tested against several important programmatic areas to examine its applicability to current problems. The examples chosen were family planning programs, dental programs for children, breast cancer screening programs and the Federal Early Periodic Screening, Diagnosis and Treatment of Children program covered by Medicaid legislation, and diabetic screening programs. These examples showed both strengths and weaknesses in the completeness of the data that were available to examine the problem.

The examination of the Early Periodic Screening, Diagnosis and Treatment Program for Children (EPSDT) under Medicaid pointed out the major deficiencies in implementation of the program, and the lack of a concentrated DHEW plan of action with regard to this program. It was concluded that this health program is typical of many that have been initiated over the past ten years by the Federal government, characterized by a relatively clear legislative mandate, a diffused administrative implementation and a negligible program commitment for research or evaluation.

The example of the mass screening programs of the American Diabetic Association showed that recent evaluation efforts have begun to lead to the conclusion that such programs are nonproductive. Isolated studies, primarily on the West Coast, have led to a major effort to change the focus of the organization and point out that the vast expenditures in time and resources could have been better utilized earlier in time had ongoing evaluation been built into such programs.

The need to improve the quality of health services, the need for accountability of health professionals in view of finite resources have resulted in recent federal legislation (PSROs) to assure that there will be continuing efforts to maintain and to upgrade the quality of health services. These efforts should be strongly supported.

In summary, this Task Force has taken the position that *there should be assessment of the adequacy of the prevalence of preventive health programs and providers and that the objectives and standards of performance of a program or a provider should be clearly enumerated. Such standards and objectives should then be periodically and systematically evaluated to assure that goals are met. Concomitantly, there should be continued application of quality controls and evaluation of standards to assure that the most effective modalities are employed to impact on the nation's health. In order to assure that these objectives are obtained, a public commitment supported by adequate program policies and funding is required.*

Recommendations

Preamble: There are continuing changes in the needs of the population, advances in the state of knowledge, and opportunities afforded through such legislation as national health insurance.

Recommendation I.

There should be continual assessment of the health problems and needs of communities and the nation as a whole in order to set priorities for introduction of or emphasis on different elements of preventive health services.

Preamble: Evaluation procedures should be developed and carried out in all programs. These should be directed at the elements outlined in the matrix in Table 1.

Recommendation II.

Penetration Rate: The target population must be defined for both primary and secondary preventive programs. Data should be obtained to measure the extent to which the program is reaching the target population and to determine the characteristics of both users and nonusers. For this purpose, commitment and long-term support for routine data systems, as well as special studies, is required.

Recommendation III.

Cost Efficiency: While costs should not be the ultimate determinant for support of effective modalities, continued review of program cost efficiency, effectiveness, and benefit should be undertaken. Continued research support should be provided to determine relative costs and efficiencies of significant components of both primary and secondary preventive health programs.

Recommendation IV.

Structure, Organization, and Financing: The effect of different types of systems on both primary and secondary preventive activities should be examined as to their relationship to program results in specific disease programs, comprehensive health care settings, hospital-based operations and solo practitioners' offices. Evaluation should also be made of the effects on program results of the method of financing; prepayment, fee-for-service, or prefunded.

Preamble: There is at this time no universally agreed upon method for the evaluation of clinical performance. All of the modalities currently in use, implicit and explicit peer review, study of process and patient outcome, clinical trials, the tracer and "critical incident method" have advantages and disadvantages depending in large measure on the existing knowledge of disease, the focus of the program or service, and amount of manpower and financial resources available.

Recommendation V.

Clinical Care: Regardless of how imperfect current measurement tools are, they are adequate to identify major flaws in health delivery and should be utilized to achieve this objective until further methodological refinements are made. Continued support should be provided to examine and develop the different methods of quality assessment.

Recommendation VI.

Support Services: Efforts to assure adequate evaluation of, and quality controls for, laboratory, x-ray, pharmacy services, and pharmaceuticals should be expanded by public agencies on both a regional and national basis. Special attention should be given to the effective use of the laboratory in preventive care. Efforts to assure accurate and precise results should include establishing local and regional quality control centers; federal licensing and certification of laboratories; and private, state and federal surveillance of actual laboratory performance.

Recommendation VII.

Health Education: Governmental action is recommended to encourage methodological research on the measurement of programs for health education and the standardization of instruments to improve the comparability of findings from various studies.

Recommendation VIII.

Reduction of Incidence: Adequate program and community wide data must be maintained and examined to determine effectiveness in reduction of incidence of disease and premature death. Data reporting systems should be carefully designed to meet objectives with minimum required input, be accurately maintained, and be compatible with other data bases.

Recommendation IX.

Health Status: Continued efforts are necessary to improve methods of classification of health status so that these indices can be utilized in a

146

variety of settings to evaluate the effectiveness of efforts in both primary and secondary prevention.

Recommendation X.

External and Internal Evaluations: Funding awards from federal and other public agencies for service and demonstration programs should include support to provide for external evaluation studies. External evaluations must be carried out: (1) to develop, demonstrate, and evaluate individual elements of prevention, e.g., testing the validity of the measurements; (2) for surveillance and monitoring to examine the extent of the effort; (3) to examine the extent to which overall community need or opportunity is met; and (4) for comparison of different modes of delivery systems.

Internal evaluation activities need to be carried out to establish the role and usefulness and effectiveness of individual elements and procedures within a program. After that has been done for an individual element of prevention, these procedures may be modified to carry out a surveillance function. Such evaluations should be built into the ongoing activities of every organized program of care and a portion of the operating budget should be allocated, adequate for this purpose, depending upon the level of the program activities.

Recommendation XI.

Long Term-Research: It is essential that long-term research be supported in the field of chronic disease to provide valid standards of care which will form the basis for ongoing evaluation efforts of primary and secondary preventive health programs.

Recommendation XII.

DHEW must accord a high priority to evaluation and quality control through the development of program policies, adequate funding and agency staffing to meet such objectives.

Recommendation XIII.

Early and substantive evaluation of the quality controls and preventive care aspects of government-sponsored programs must be undertaken.

Recommendation XIV.

The PSRO effort must be supported and selected local agencies permitted to vary their approaches to both quality and utilization review

147

until relative effectiveness of different approaches is demonstrated. Financial support for data collection and analysis should be provided on an on-going basis. Review of preventive health services and ambulatory care should be introduced as rapidly as possible.

Evaluation Study Examples

Subject: *Family Planning Programs*

Primary Prevention. Preventing unwanted pregnancies by contraceptive methods.

Secondary Prevention. Provision of clinic and support services for: (1) unwanted pregnancies (abortion or prenatal care); (2) wanted pregnancies (infertility services and prenatal care).

Nature of the Problem. It was estimated in 1973 that 1.9 million low-income and 1.8 million marginal income women at risk were still apparently without access to effective modern methods of contraception[141] even though the overall crude birthrate declined by more than 41 percent and the general fertility rate declined by 44 percent[142] between the years 1957 and 1973. The Secretary of HEW has given major credit for this decline to the federal family planning efforts. "By reducing unwanted births, the program has been cost effective, saving more than two dollars for every dollar spent."[143]

Summary. Major evaluation enforts in family planning have been directed at the areas of penetration rate, cost effectiveness, effectiveness of the methods employed, and the obvious outcome in terms of fewer pregnancies. There is, however, a dearth of evaluation of quality of clinical process and performance (Table 7).

General References

A.A. Campbell, "The Role of Family Planning in the Reduction of Poverty," *Journal of Marriage and the Family* 30:236, 1968.

Patricia K. Chokel and Janet T. Dingle, "Using Standard Data for Program Evaluation in Cleveland," *Family Planning Perspectives* 4:216, 1973.

Hector Correa, Vestal W. Parrish, Jr., and Joseph D. Beasley, "A Three-Year Longitudinal Evaluation of the Costs of a Family Planning Program," *American Journal of Public Health* 12:1647, 1972.

Committee on Terminology of the National Family Planning Forum, "A Family Planning Glossary," *Family Planning Perspectives,* 3:34, 1972.

Charles R. Dean, "Staffing Patterns and Clinic Efficiency," *Family Planning Perspectives,* 4:35, 1970.

Steven Polgar and Frederick S. Jaffe, "Evaluation and Record-keeping for the U.S. Family Planning Services," *Public Health Reports,* 8:639, 1968.

Steven Polgar, O. Ornati, and J.G. Dryfoos, "How to Estimate Unmet Need for Family Planning in Your Community," *American Journal of Public Health,* 56:917, 1966.

Table 7. Evaluation of Family Planning Programs

Evaluation Element: Penetration Rate
Example of Data Needed and/or Applicable Methods and Results: In the United States, in 1973, it was estimated that 5.6 million low-income and an additional 3.4 million marginal income women needed family planning services. Of these, 65 percent received services from either organized programs or private physicians.[1]

Evaluation Element: Cost Efficiency
Example of Data Needed and/or Applicable Methods and Results: The National Analyst study collected cost data on 45 family planning projects for the program year of 1968–1969 utilizing cost line items and service categories for collection and analysis of the cost data. It was determined that "the per patient cost to the average project for the year 1968–1969 was about $76. If the total operating cost of the 45 projects for the same year was divided by the total number of women seen at least once during the year, an annual unit cost per patient was about $53."[2]

Evaluation Element: Structure and Organization
Example of Data Needed and/or Applicable Methods and Results: In addition to a review of the facilities, scope of services, administrative organization, etc., evaluation of staffing patterns and patient/staff ratios can be carried out. One example of this is Perkins's Patient/Staff Index.[3] By using this particular evaluative measure, it was found that clinics whose staffs were fully utilized during a session reported a higher patient/staff index than clinics which were either over-staffed or under-utilized. It was also found that clinics which report an unusually high index potentially were not providing adequate individual patient care or were requiring existing staff to process too many patients during a single session.

Evaluation Element: Process Modalities—Clinical, Laboratory, and X-ray
Example of Data Needed and/or Applicable Methods and Results: Family planning care standards and criteria have been established by such groups as the ACOG and Maternal and Infant Care-Family Planning Programs. However, there has not been extensive evaluation of care against these standards and criteria.

Evaluation Element: Process Modalities—Health Education
Example of Data Needed and/or Applicable Methods and Results: Planned Parenthood of Buffalo was involved in the production of TV spots and in the follow-up studies of their effectiveness. Each set of TV spots carried a different phone number to call for information, to be able to measure the general responses as well as to find out which spot was most appealing. The effectiveness was judged significant in that 51 percent or approximately every other person who called during the two month period, made and kept an appointment.[4]

Evaluation Element: Program Results—Reduction of Incidence
Example of Data Needed and/or Applicable Methods and Results: Determination of reduction of incidence of pregnancies requires data collection and analysis of birth rate changes, etc., utilizing such sources as census data, birth certificates, hospital delivery figures. For example, in Atlanta, Georgia, a study was done to see if there was any effect from the family planning program at Grady Memorial Hospital. The clinic enrollment had doubled from 1963 to 1968 and during this same period, births at the hospital declined from 7,125 a year to 5,935—a decrease of 17 percent.[5]

Evaluation Element: Program Results—Health Status
Example of Data Needed and/or Applicable Methods and Results: Though implications have been made concerning the effect/benefit of family planning on such areas as housing availability, poverty levels, numbers within the educational systems and an increased female work force[6] as well as improved marital adjustment and less child abuse, little evaluative research has been carried out in this area.

[1] Marsha Corey, "The State of Organized Family Planning Programs in the United States, 1973," *Family Planning Perspectives* 1:15, 1974.

[2] Gerald Sparer, Louise Okada, and Stanley Tillinghast, "How Much Do Family Planning Programs Cost?", *Family Planning Perspectives* 2:100, 1973.

[3] Gordon W. Perkins, "Measuring Clinic Performance," *Family Planning Perspectives* 1:37, 1969.

[4] Jean Hutchinson, "Using TV to Recruit Family Planning Patients," *Family Planning Perspectives* 2:8, 1970.

[5] Carl W. Taylor et al., "Assessment of a Family Planning Program: Contraceptive Services and Fertility in Atlanta, Georgia," *Family Planning Perspectives* 2:25, 1970.

[6] James A. Sweet, "Differentials in the Rate of Fertility Decline 1960–1970," *Family Planning Perspectives* 2:103, 1974.

Michael J. Reardon et al. "Real Costs of Delivering Family Planning Services— Implications for Management," *American Journal of Public Health,* 9:860, 1974.

M. Tayback, "Evaluation of Family Planning Programs," Paper presented at the Institute in Administration of New Programs in Maternal and Child Health, University of California, Berkeley, January 19, 1966.

Subject: Dental Programs for Children

Primary Prevention. Prevention of dental disease, abnormalities, and injury to and loss of dental and surrounding oral structures.

Secondary prevention. Correction of hereditary and congenital defects and defects caused by dental disease. Slowing progress of dental disease and limiting its extent.

Nature of the Problem. Based on examinations, approximately 24 million U.S. children aged 6–11 years averaged an estimated 1.4 DMF teeth per child. The estimate consists of 0.5 decayed, 0.1 missing, and 0.8 filled permanent teeth. As classified by the periodontal index, an estimated 9.2 million children or about 39 percent of the population aged 6–11 years, had either gingival inflammation or a more advanced form of periodontal disease. Faulty oral hygiene, due primarily to the presence of soft foreign material loosely attached to teeth, was highly prevalent among U.S. children, i.e., two-thirds had moderate to heavy debris.[148,149]

Summary. "With the increased interest in quality of dental care, more intensive evaluative efforts must be undertaken. . . . Evaluations can be considered within a framework that encompasses four levels of concern: specific activity, oral cavity, person, and group; and four dimensions of resources: technical, logistical, organizational, and financial. Evaluations can be performed as self or peer reviews or can be carried out by persons other than dentists or other dental staff members. These evaluations can be accomplished in a variety of ways, including, but not limited to, observing performances, examining, interviewing, and questioning patients and providers, inspecting facilities, and reviewing patient charts, radiographs and other sources of information . . . there have been some, albeit too few, research endeavors to formulate overall methodologies, develop specific indexes and standards, test various methods of evaluation, and determine the consequences of dental care on oral and general health and wellbeing."[150] See Table 8.

151

Table 8.   Evaluation of Dental Programs for Children

Evaluation Element: Penetration Rate
Example of Data Needed and/or Applicable Methods and Results: In 1965, the Division of Health Examination Statistics concluded a Health Survey of children aged 6-11 years which included a dental examination. The target population totaled approximately 24 million children with the sample consisting of 7,417 children. Of these 7,417 children, 7,109 received a dental examination, a 95.8 sample penetration rate.[1]

Evaluation Element: Cost Efficiency
Example of Data Needed and/or Applicable Methods and Results: The following is used as an example, though adults are also a part of the population base. On the premise that prevention and control of dental disease at an early age and for a lifetime will cause a substantial reduction in treatment expenditures, estimates of the reductions in dental expenditures were developed. Total statewide (Iowa) expenditures were estimated from the mean gross income of Iowa dentists ($51,453) multiplied by the number of dentists (about 1,220). This total ($62,772,660) was then divided by the Iowa population (2,825,041) reported by the Bureau of Census. The per capita expenditure for all dental services was estimated at $22.20. This per capita expenditure was then subdivided into expenditures for each type of dental service received and the percent reduction in expenditures from various preventive procedures estimated for each dental service. It was estimated that "if the patient were to visit a prevention-oriented dentist regularly and practice effective home care, he would be able to reduce his dental expenditures from $22.20 to $14.30 a year, or from $1,554 to $1,001 in a lifetime; this represents a 36 percent savings."[2]

Evaluation Element: Structure and Organization
Example of Data Needed and/or Applicable Methods and Results: The "Friedman system" contains a Dental Care Index which evaluates a dental care program's organizational features; extent of coverage (eligibility); scope of benefits and administrative provisions to assure quality of dental care.[3,4]

Evaluation Element: Process Modalities—Clinical, Laboratory and X-ray: Example of Data Needed and/or Applicable Methods and Results: One reliable and accurate approach to evaluation of quality of operator performance is the use of clinical examination of children under care or who have completed treatment. In dentistry, the area involved is open to direct inspection. Very little time or patient inconvenience is required to verify original diagnosis, treatment plan and treatment provided. The evidence of dental treatment and quality of performance is not only evident at the time of care but weeks, months and years later.[5] An example of the process of evaluation by dental examiners is described in Vital and Health Statistics Series 1, No. 10. Chart audit, either using the index approach and/or the peer review approach, based on explicit criteria can also be used. In one study, 15 NHC programs were reviewed between May 1971 and June 1972.[6] One of the peer review findings was that the ratings for preventive care were among the lowest components in this phase. Numerous other approaches to dental care evaluation are being used, including: Schonfeld's,[7] Clark's,[8] Cons's[9] and the Indian Health Service.[10]

Evaluation Element: Process Modalities—Health Education
Example of Data Needed and/or Applicable Methods and Results: It is comparatively easy to evaluate effectiveness of dental education, oral hygiene instruction, diet, habit control, etc., for the dental patient since results are readily detectable and quantifiable with a high degree of accuracy. The use of oral hygiene indices, DMF, d e f, malocclusion indices, etc. gives the evaluator tools to judge performance of provider (and consumer) and effectiveness of dental programs.[5]

Evaluation Element: Program Results—Reduction of Incidence and Health Status
Example of Data Needed and/or Applicable Methods and Results: A study was carried out on children eligible for service at the group practice part of the ILWU-PMA program in the Los Angeles harbor area. The study tool, originally developed by Knutson in 1938, is based on the fact that "in children, the first molar is the permanent tooth most frequently extracted for reasons of disease. It is rarely congenitally missing, or extracted for orthodontic reasons. Therefore, a rapid and inexpensive study of the tooth-saving effect of a children's dental care program can be based on the mortality of the first permanent molar."[11] Of the 1,140 children in the study, 96 percent were followed over a nine and a half

year period. Excluding congenitally missing teeth and teeth extracted for orthodontic reasons, the number of teeth missing decreased from 0.39 per child for those who became 15 years old in the first study period to 0.05 per child for those who became 15 after having been in the program for approximately nine years.

[1] National Center for Health Statistics: Periodontal Disease and Oral Hygiene Among Children. Vital and Health Statistics. Series 11, No. 117 DHEW Pub. No. (HSM) 72-1060. Washington, U.S. Government Printing Office, June, 1972.

[2] Raymond F. Falasco and William G. Henderson, "Estimated Reduction in Dental Expenditures for Iowans through Preventive Programs," *J. Amer. Dental Assoc.* Vol. 86:627, 1973.

[3] H.K. Schonfeld, "Dental Evaluation Systems in the United States," *Public Health Reviews.* 4:403, 1974.

[4] J.W. Friedman, *The Dental Care Index: A Systematic Approach to the Evaluation of Dental Care Programs.* Supported under a grant provided by the National Institutes of Health at the U.C.L.A. School of Public Health.

[5] Leon Lewis, D.D.S., Personal communication.

[6] Walter Wolford, Mildred Morehead, and Rose Donaldson, "Quality of Dental Care in Ambulatory Care Centers," Presented at the Dental Health Session, APHA, Atlantic City, N.J., 1972.

[7] H.K. Schonfeld et al. "The Content of Good Dental Care: Methodology in a Formulation for Clinical Standards and Audits, and Preliminary Findings," *AJPH.* 7:1137, July, 1967.

[8] C.C. Clark et al, "Evaluation of a Dental Care Program," *Health Service Report.* 88:763, 1973.

[9] N.C. Cons, "The Clinical Evaluation of Medicaid's Patients in the State of New York," *J. Pub. Health Dent.* 33:186, 1973.

[10] Indian Health Service, Dental Services Branch, *Quality of Dental Care Evaluation System ftr the Indian Health Service.* U.S. DHEW, PHS, HSMHA, Washington, D.C. 1972.

[11] Max Schoen, "Effect of a Prepaid Children's Dental Program on Mortality of Permanent Teeth," *J. Amer. Dental Assoc.* Vol. 71:626, 1965.

Subject: Breast Cancer Screening Programs

Primary Prevention.   None.

Secondary Prevention.   Reduction of breast cancer mortality.

Nature of the Problem.   Breast cancer mortality among women has remained unchanged in the United States for over 40 years; it is the leading cause of death from cancer of many adults in the female population.

Summary.   Screening with mammography and clinical examinations on a one or two year reexamination cycle for women 50 years of age or older appears to be a reasonable immediate preventive health program advisable for widespread application. The issue of efficacy of routine mammography in asymptomatic women in the 35 to 50 age range is still in question and additional studies are needed to resolve the question.

Other issues requiring further research include periodicity; annual versus biennial screening; lowest age for screening programs; use of nonphysicians for preliminary screening of x-ray films and for physical examination of the breast; reduction in the amount of radiation dosage required, and high-risk factors. See Table 9.

Table 9. Evelution of Breast Cancer Screening Programs

Evaluation Element: Penetration Rate

Example of Data Needed and/or Applicable Methods and Results: Penetration rates should be based on the proportion of the target population that participates in the initial screening examination and in successive reexaminations. For example, in the HIP randomized controlled trial in New York, 31,000 women aged 40–64 years were offered screening by both palpation and mammography. Of these, 20,211 or 65 percent had an initial screening examination.[1] Characteristics of participants and nonparticipants should be studied as in the HIP studies, with activities developed to reduce nonparticipation.[1,2]

Evaluation Element: Cost Efficiency

Example of Data Needed and/or Applicable Methods and Results: Analysis can be carried out on the dollar costs per screening examination and per breast cancer case detected; total costs to be broken down by nonmedical expenditures for educational programs, communication with target population, follow-up of positive cases; personnel costs for clinical and radiologic examination; administrative and equipment costs. Man-hours (technical and medical) per screening examination should be computed, classifying input by type of personnel and activity.

Evaluation Element: Structure and Organization

Example of Data Needed and/or Applicable Methods and Results: Review of the general organizational aspects of a program and staff; qualifications of the personnel. If the personnel are nonphysicians, the content of their training should be reviewed. Mechanisms for follow-up, screening false positives and referral for treatment should be examined for efficacy.

Evaluation Element: Process Modalities—Clinical, X-ray, Thermography

Example of Data Needed and/or Applicable Methods and Results: Analysis of the effectiveness of various detection methods, e.g., palpation, mammography and thermography. For example, the HIP study showed that of the cases discovered at screening, 22 percent were detected by both palpation and mammography, 45 percent by palpation alone and 33 percent by mammography alone.[3] New experience is being accumulated by the NCI/ACS breast cancer detection project in 27 centers and involving over a quarter of a million women. The value of thermography is being assessed for screening.

Performance of staff in breast examinations and mammographic interpretation reviewed for quality and accuracy; as well as evaluation of the quality of films, radiation exposure and protection against scatter to other organs of the body.

Evaluation Element: Process Modalities—Health Education

Example of Data Needed and/or Applicable Methods and Results: Extensive efforts utilizing repeat mailing and telephone calls required in the HIP study to increase participation rates from two out of five to two out of three.

Evaluation Element: Program Results

Example of Data Needed and/or Applicable Methods and Results: Results of a large randomized clinical trial (HIP) indicated that periodic screening for breast cancer leads to a short-run reduction of close to a third in mortality from this condition.[4] Follow-up has covered a seven-year period; longer periods of follow-up are needed to determine the persistence of the benefit. Reduction in breast cancer mortality in the study under way has been limited to women 50 years of age and older; no reduction is evidenced under 50.

---

[1] Raymond Fink, Sam Shapiro, and Ruth Roester, "Impact of Efforts to Increase Participation in Repetitive Screenings for Early Breast Cancer Detection," *AJPH.* 62:328, March 1972.

[2] Raymond Fink, Sam Shapiro, and John Lewison. "The Reluctant Participant in a Breast Cancer Screening Program," *Public Health Reports.* 6:479, 1968.

[3] S. Shapiro, P. Strax, I. Venet, and M. Venet, *Changes in 5-Year Breast Cancer Mortality in a Breast Cancer Screening Program.* 7th National Cancer Conference. J. B. Lippincott Co., Philadelphia, pp. 663–678.

[4] S. Shapiro, "Screening for Early Detection of Cancer and Heart Disease," *Bulletin of the New York Academy of Medicine,* 1:80, January 1975.

Subject: *Early Periodic Screening, Diagnosis and Treatment (EPSDT) — Medicaid*

Primary Prevention. Evaluate each child to determine unmet need for services and to provide primary preventive services and health supervision.

Secondary Prevention. Provide treatment and referral for problems identified.

Nature of the Problem. In 1967, amendments to Title XIX of the Social Security Act mandated reaching the high-risk, high-priority children in needy families. Expectation was for implementation of the program by July of 1969. Reports [151,152] indicate major deficiencies in program implementation. General Accounting Office (GAO) estimates that it is working in probably no more than six to eight states, while in over 40 states it is not working at all. Problems are "lack of funds and lack of providers." From an administrative standpoint, major problems can be attributed to the lack of departmental commitment and capacity to implement the program. In June of 1972, after four and one-half years and pressure from such groups as the National Welfare Rights Organization, the Medical Services Administration (MSA) issued guidelines for the program. Following that, Social and Rehabilitation Services (SRS), in cooperation with the American Academy of Pediatrics, issued guidelines and an evaluation handbook for the EPSDT model which were issued in September of 1974. Social and Rehabilitation Services and MSA have primarily limited their activities to issuing guidelines. As yet, it is difficult to discern a concentrated DHEW plan of action with regard to this program.

This health program is typical of many that have been initiated over the past ten years, characterized by a relatively clear legislative mandate, a diffused administrative implementation and an almost nonexistent program commitment for research or evaluation.

Summary. What is needed is an updated national study outlining the degree of implementation of the EPSDT program. Additional evaluation could include the relative yield from the screening activities to positive diagnosis and follow-up treatment. Additional research should be undertaken to document the efficacy of screening relative to treatment related to health outcome objectives. Evaluation could be carried out of alternate models for screening and treatment via the school health programs at elementary, junior high, and high school levels including a pregraduation screening. Examination of the relative productivity of procedures should also be undertaken so that the most efficient models for the program can be implemented in states with minimal budget capacity. See Table 10.

Table 10. Evaluation of Early Periodic Screening, Diagnosis, and Treatment of Children

Evaluation Element: Penetration Rate

Example of Data Needed and/or Applicable Methods and Results: The base against which penetration efforts were to be measured were Medicaid-eligible children within a specific jurisdiction (census tract, precinct, borough, county, etc.) for which the EPSDT demonstration activity had area/population jurisdiction.[1] In all, it was estimated that approximately ten million children would have been eligible to EPSDT or 12 percent of the U.S. child population of 80 million.[2] Reportedly, one million have been screened (AFDC, APTD, AB).[3]

Evaluation Element: Cost Efficiency

Example of Data Needed and/or Applicable Methods and Results: In the Demonstration Model Evaluation Handbook for the EPSDT program,[1] it was suggested that a cost analysis be done in such areas as: cost per test; cost per outreach by method; cost of referral and follow-up; rate of confirmed findings (well and unwell) per average cost per screen; and rate of conversion (unwell to well) per average cost per case for diagnosis and treatment.

Evaluation Element: Structure and Organization

Example of Data Needed and/or Applicable Methods and Results: The Guidelines were published by DHEW-SRSV/MSA in June of 1972.[4] A study[5] was conducted in the winter through summer of 1972 to determine the extent to which the Title XIX program was being implemented, areas where progress had been made and to identify problems needing attention. A study form was sent to State Maternal and Child Health and Crippled Children's Program Directors and to State Welfare Departments. Complete replies were received from 44 of the 54 states and territories and partial replies from six states. Thirty-eight of the respondents reported provision of health care for children under Title XIX. Of the 44 complete respondent states, 19 reported that standards had been established.

Evaluation Element: Process Modalities—Clinical, Laboratory, and X-ray

Example of Data Needed and/or Applicable Methods and Results: In June of 1974, "A Guide to Screening for the EPSDT Program under Medicaid" was developed by the SRS in cooperation with the American Academy of Pediatrics.[6] The extent of implementation and evaluation of care in relation to them is unknown.

The Evaluation Handbook (September, 1974)[3] suggested that a professional review board do a 15 percent sample of the same children with the same tests and equipment to establish an independent rate of functional accuracy which would be used to determine a rate of confirmed findings relative to the demonstration screening team's findings. No results have been reported on this yet.

Evaluation Element: Process Modalities—Health Education

Example of Data Needed and/or Applicable Methods and Results: Information not available.

Evaluation Element: Program Results—Reduction of Incidence and Health Status

Example of Data Needed and/or Applicable Methods and Results: It was planned (Evaluation Handbook)[1] that the studies would measure change in the target population over time in the following conditions or areas: (1) the general status of child health through means of a healthiness rating; (2) immunization status; (3) seriousness and type of disease/injury condition; (4) utilization of various community health services and (5) Medicaid costs. In addition, special studies were planned on recipient attitude, staff and provider attitude. To date, no results have been reported.

---

[1] Regional Health Services Research Institute. *EPSDT-Demonstration Model Evaluation Handbook.* University of Texas Health Science Center, San Antonio, Texas. September 1, 1974. have be

[2] Ann-Marie Foltz, "The Development of Ambiguous Federal Policy: Early and Periodic Screening, Diagnosis and Treatment (EPSDT)," *The Milbank Memorial Fund Quarterly, Health and Society.* 1:35, Winter, 1975.

[3] Gerald Sparer, Acting Director, Division of Health Services Evaluation, National Center for Health Services Research, Public Health Service, DHEW. Personal Communication.

[4] *Early and Periodic Screening Diagnosis-Treatment-For Individuals Under 21 (Medicaid)—Guidelines.* U.S. DHEW, Social and Rehabilitation Service and Medical Services Administration.

[5] Helen M. Wallace, Hyman Goldstein, and Allan C. Oglesby, "The Health and Medical Care of Children under Title XIX Medicaid," *AJPH* 5:501, 1974.

[6] William K. Frankenburg, and A. Frederick North, *A Guide to Screening For the Early and Periodic Screening, Diagnosis and Treatment Program (EPSDT) under Medicaid.* Prepared by the American Academy of Pediatrics under Contract SRS 73-31, Social and Rehabilitation Service, U.S. DHEW.

References

[1] Mindel C. Sheps, "Approaches to the Quality of Hospital Care," *Public Health Rep.* 70:877, September, 1955.

[2] Mindel C. Sheps, "Assessing Effectiveness of Programs in Operation," Fourth Conference on Administrative Medicine, 1955, *Transactions*, p. 111–124, Josiah Macy, Jr., Foundation, 1956.

[3] H.B. Makover, "The Quality of Medical Care: Methodological Survey of the Medical Groups Associated with the Health Insurance Plan of New York," *American Journal of Public Health*, 46:848, 1956.

[4] R.E. Trussel, M.A. Morehead, J. Ehrlich, et al., *The Quantity, Quality and Costs of Medical and Hospital Care Secured by a Sample of Teamster Families in the New York Area*, Columbia University School of Public Health and Administrative Medicine, 1962.

[5] M.A. Morehead, and R. Donaldson, "Quality of Clinical Management of Disease in Comprehensive Neighborhood Health Centers," *Medical Care* 4:301, 1974.

[6] F.M. Richardon, "Peer Review of Medical Care," *Medical Care* 1:29, 1972.

[7] M.A. Morehead et al., *A Study of the Quality of Hospital Care Secured by a Sample of Teamster Family Members in New York City*, Columbia University School of Public Health and Administrative Medicine, 1964.

[8] L.S. Rosenfeld, "Quality of Medical Care in Hospitals," *American Journal of Public Health* 47:856, 1957.

[9] Beverly C. Payne, "Continued Evolution of a System of Medical Care Appraised," *Journal of the American Medical Association* 7:126, 1967.

[10] Office of Professional Standards Review, *PSRO Program Manual*, DHEW, 1974.

[11] P.A. Lembcke, "A Scientific Method for Medical Auditing," *Hospitals* 33: part 1, 65–71; part 2, 65–72, 1959.

[12] Office of Community Health Centers, *Approaches to Quality of Care Assessment*, Bureau of Community Health Services, Health Services Administration, DHEW, 1975.

[13] Sheldon Greenfield, Personal communication, 1975.

[14] E.A. Codman, "The Product of a Hospital," *Surg. Gynec. Obstet.* 18:491, 1914.

[15] Paul A. Lembcke, "Evolution of the Medical Audit," *Journal of the American Medical Association* 8:111, 1967.

[16] Paul J. Sanazaro, and John W. Williamson, "End Results of Patient Care: A Provisional Classification Based on Reports by Internists," *Medical Care* 2:123, 1968.

[17] Willy DeGeyndt, *A Tentative Framework for the Evaluation of the Children and Youth Program*, Paper presented at the June 17, 1969 Children and Youth Evaluation Conference sponsored by the Systems Development Project and supported by a grant from the United States Children's Bureau.

[18] John W. Williamson, "Evaluating Quality of Patient Care—A Strategy Relating Outcome and Process Assessment," *JAMA* 4:564, 1971.

[19] Joseph Gonnella, and Carter Zeleznik, "Factors Involved in Comprehensive Patient Care Evaluation," *Medical Care* 11:928, 1974.

[20] Avedis Donabedian, *A Perspective on Concepts of Health Care Quality,* Paper given at the New York Academy of Medicine's Annual Health Conference on the Professional Responsibility for Quality of Health Care, April 24, 1975.

[21] George B. Hutchison, "Evaluation of Preventive Services," *Journal of Chronic Diseases* 5:497, 1960.

[22] Arlene Barro, "Survey and Evaluation of Approaches to Physician Performance Measurement," *Journal of Medical Education* 48:1051, 1973.

[23] John W. Williamson, Personal communication.

[24] Samuel B. Hagner, Victor J. LoCicero, and William A. Steiger. "Patient Outcome in a Comprehensive Medicine Clinic: Its Retrospective Assessment and Related Variables," *Medical Care* 2:144, 1968.

[25] John W. Williamson, "Outcomes of Health Care: Key to Health Improvement," *Outcomes Conference I-II: Methodology of Identifying and Evaluating Outcomes of Health Service Programs, Systems and Subsystems,* Rockville, Maryland: U.S. Department of Health, Education, and Welfare, National Center for Health Services Research and Development, 1969, p. 75.

[26] Veterans Administration Study Group on Antihypertensive Agents, "Effects of treatment on morbidity in hypertension. I. Results in patients with diastolic blood pressure averaging 115 through 129 mm Hg," *JAMA.* 202:1028–1034, 1967. "II. Results in patients with diastolic blood pressure averaging 90 through 114 mm Hg," *JAMA.* 213:1143–1152, 1970.

[27] Barbara Starfield.

[28] "Behavioral Factors Associated with the Etiology of Physical Disease," (includes six papers) *AJPH,* 11:1033, 1974.

[29] N.Q. Brill, et. al., "Controlled Study of Psychiatric Outpatient Treatment," *Archives of General Psychiatry,* 10:581, 1964.

[30] D.M. Kessner, C.E. Kalk, and J. Singer, "Assessing Health Quality—The Case for Tracers," *New England Journal of Medicine* 288:189–194, 1973.

[31] D.M. Kessner, J. Singer, C.E. Kalk, and E.R. Schlesinger, *Infant Death: An Analysis by Maternal Risk and Health Care. Contrasts in Health Status,* Vol. 1. Washington, D.C.: National Academy of Sciences, 1973.

[32] D.M. Kessner and C.E. Kalk, *A Strategy for Evaluating Health Services, Contrasts in Health Status,* Vol. 2. Washington, D.C.: National Academy of Sciences, 1973.

[33] D.M. Kessner, C.K. Snow, and J. Singer, *Assessment of Medical Care for Children. Contrasts in Health Status,* Vol. 3. Washington, D.C.: National Academy of Sciences, 1974.

[34] National Academy of Sciences, Institute of Medicine, Health Services Research Study. *Development of Methodology for Evaluation of Neighborhood Health Centers.* Prepared for United States Department of Health, Education, and Welfare, Office of Deputy Assistant Secretary of Evaluation and Monitoring, Health Evaluation Office (Contract No. HEW-OS-70-130), Washington, D.C., 1972. Available through National Technical Information Service, Springfield, Virginia as PB-213-314.

[35] Albert Einstein College of Medicine, Department of Community Health, Evaluation Unit, *Ambulatory Health Care Services Review Manual.* Pursuant to Grant 2812A from Division

of Program Planning and Evaluation, Office for Health Affairs, Office of Economic Opportunity, n.d.

[36] A. Donabedian, "Promoting Quality through Evaluating the Process of Patient Care," *Medical Care* VI:181–202, 1968.

[37] M.E.W. Goss, G.G. Reader, O.S. Ochs, M.H. Mushinski, and J.E. Brewin, *Toward an Evaluation Framework for Neighborhood Health Centers.* Final Report for Community Health Service, Health Services and Mental Health Administration (Grant No. CS-H-000002-01-0), New York, N.Y., 1972. Available through National Technical Information Service, Springfield, Virginia, as PB-233-574/HS.

[38] J.H. Langston et al., *Study to Evaluate the OEO Neighborhood Health Center Program at Selected Centers.* Final Report for Office of Economic Opportunity (Contract No. B00-5104), GEOMET Report No. HF-71, Rockville, Md., 1972.

[39] M.A. Morehead, R.S. Donaldson, and M.R. Seravalli, "Comparisons between OEO Neighborhood Health Centers and Other Health Care Providers of Ratings of the Quality of Health Care," *American Journal of Public Health* 61:1294–1306, 1971.

[40] M.I. Roemer, "Evaluation of Health Service Programs and Levels of Measurements," *HSMHA Health Reports* 86:839–848, 1971.

[41] S. Shapiro, "End Result Measurements of Quality of Medical Care," *Milbank Memorial Fund Quarterly* XLV:7–30, 1967.

[42] G. Sparer, and J. Johnson, "Evaluation of OEO Neighborhood Health Centers," *American Journal of Public Health* 61:931–942, 1971.

[43] V.E. Weckwerth, *Progress Report: Assessment of Child Health Care Delivery and Organization,* University of Minnesota, Systems Development Project COMMENT SERIES No. 0-7 (29), April 1970.

[44] Joseph S. Gonnella, Daniel Z. Louis, and John J. McCord, *An Approach to the Assessment of Outcome of Ambulatory Care* Presented at the Joint Meeting of the Operations Research Society of America and the Institute of Management Sciences, San Juan, Puerto Rico, October 16, 1974.

[45] J.C. Hershey, "Consequence Evaluation in Decision Analytic Models of Medical Screening, Diagnosis, and Treatment," *Methods of Information in Medicine* 13 (4):197, 1974.

[46] D.A.B. Lindberg and R.R. Watson, "Imprecision of Laboratory Determinations and Diagnostic Accuracy; Theoretical Considerations," *Methods of Information in Medicine* 13 (3):151, 1974.

[47] *Principles and Practice of Screening for Disease,* Technical Report No. 34, World Health Organization.

[48] *Mass Health Examination,* Technical Report No. 45, World Health Organization.

[49] System Sciences, Inc. *Preliminary Report on Cost-Effectiveness of Urine Testing,* Prepared for National Institute on Drug Abuse, Department of Health, Education, and Welfare, November 1974.

[50] L.W. Green, "Toward Cost-Benefit Evaluations of Health Education: Some Concepts, Methods and Examples," *Health Education Monographs* 2 (Supplement No. 1): 34–60, May 1974.

159

[51] L.W. Green and I. Figa-Talamanca, "Suggested Designs for Evaluation of Health Education Programs," *Health Education Monographs* 2:54–71, Spring 1974.

[52] L.W. Green, D.M. Levine, and S. Deeds, *Clinical Trials of Health Education for Hypertensive Outpatients: Design and Baseline Data,* Paper presented at the Eastern Section of the American Federation for Clinical Research, January 1975.

[53] L.W. Green, "Cost Containment and the Economics of Health Education in Medical Care," *Hospitals, J.A.H.A.* 49: in press, 1975.

[54] A.G. Oetlinger and N. Zapol, "Will Information Technologies Help Learning?" *Teachers College Record* 74:5–54, September 1972.

[55] L.W. Green, "Diffusion and Adoption of Innovations Related to Cardiovascular Risk Behavior in the Public," in C. Enelow, J. Henderson, and E. Berkanovic, (eds.), *Applying Behavioral Sciences to Cardiovascular Risk,* New York: American Heart Association, 1975.

[56] P.L. Campeau, "Selective Review of the Results of Research on the Use of Audiovisual Media to Teach Adults," *AV Communications Review* 22:5–40, Spring 1974.

[57] S.G. Deeds, "Promises! Promises! Educational Technology for Health Education Audiences," Presented at the American Public Health Association, San Francisco, 1973.

[58] S.R. Fletcher, *A Study of the Effectiveness of a Follow-Up Clerk in an Emergency Room,* Unpublished Master of Science Thesis, Baltimore: Johns Hopkins University School of Hygiene and Public Health, 1973.

[59] J.B. Atwater, "Adapting the Venereal Disease Clinic to Today's Problems," *American Journal of Public Health* 64:433–437, May 1974.

[60] W.R. Cuskey and T. Prekumer, "A differential Role Model for the Treatment of Drug Addicts," *Health Services Reports* 88:663–668, 1973.

[61] D.M. Tagliacozzo et al., "Nurse Intervention and Patient Behavior: An Experimental Study," *American Journal of Public Health* 64:596–603, June 1974.

[62] S.P. Rosenzweig and R. Folman, "Patient and Therapist Variables Affecting Premature Termination in Group Psychotherapy," *Psychotherapy: Theory, Research and Practice* 11:76–79, Spring 1974.

[63] B. Freemon et al., "Gaps in Doctor-Patient Communications: Doctor-Patient Interaction Analysis," *Pediatric Research* 5:298–311, 1971.

[64] L.W. Green, "Should Health Education Abandon Attitude Change Strategies: Perspectives from Recent Research," *Health Education Monographs* 1(30):25–48, 1970.

[65] E.L. Baker and M.C. Alkin, "ERIC/AVCR Annual Review Paper: Formative Evaluation of Instructional Development," *AV Communication Review* 21:389–418, Winter 1973.

[66] M.H. Becker, (ed.), "Personal Health Practices and the Health Belief Model," *Health Education Monographs* 2:324–473, Winter 1974.

[67] R.B. Cattell, "How Good is the Modern Questionnaire? General Principles of Evaluation," *Journal of Personality Assessment* 38:115–129, April 1974.

[68] G.M. Maranell, (ed.), *Scaling: A Sourcebook for Behavioral Scientists,* Chicago: Aldine, 1974.

[69] J. Schopler et al., "The North Carolina Internal-External Scale: Validation of the Short Form," *Research Previews* 20:3–12, November 1973.

[70] L. Mezei: "Factorial Validity of the Kluckhohn and Strodtbeck Value Orientation Scale," *Journal of Social Psychology* 92:145–146, February 1974.

[71] L.W. Green: *Status Identity and Preventive Health Behavior,* Berkeley: University of California, Pacific Health Education Reports No. 1, 1970.

[72] L.W. Green: Manual for Scoring Socioeconomic Status for Research on Health Behavior," *Public Health Reports* 85:815–827, September 1970.

[73] D. Coburn and Clyde R. Pope: "Socioeconomic Status and Preventive Health Behavior," *Journal of Health and Social Behavior* 15:67–78, June 1974.

[74] J. Saunders, J.M. Davis, and D.M. Monsees: "Opinion Leadership in Family Planning," *Journal of Health and Social Behavior* 15:217–227, September 1974.

[75] A.A. Fisher: "The Predictive Validity of a Measure of Opinion Leadership in Family Planning," *Health Education Monographs* 3: in press, Summer 1975.

[76] R.L. Stevenson: "Cross-Cultural Validation of a Readership Prediction Technique," *Journalism Quarterly* 50:690–696, Winter 1973.

[77] F.B. Collen and K. Soghikian: "Health Exhibits Accentuate the Positive," *Hospitals, J.A.H.A.* 48:92–95, March 16, 1974.

[78] J.A. Czepiel: "Word-of-Mouth Processes in the Diffusion of a Major Technological Innovation," *Journal of Marketing Research* 11:172–180, May 1974.

[79] J.R. Lynn: "Perception of Public Service Advertising: Source, Message and Receiver Effects," *Journalism Quarterly* 50:673–679, 689, Winter 1973.

[80] A.W. Thornton: "Mass Communications and Dental Health Behavior," *Health Education Monographs* 2:201–208, Fall 1974.

[81] J.N. Kerri: "Anthropological Studies of Voluntary Associations and Voluntary Action: A Review," *Journal of Voluntary Action Research* 3:10–25, January 1974.

[82] P.E. White and G.T. Vlasak: *Interorganizational Research in Health: Bibliography (1960–70),* Washington: U.S. Dept. of Health, Education, and Welfare, DHEW Pub. (HSM) 72-3,028,1972.

[83] J.M. Metsch and J.E. Veney: "Measuring the Outcome of Consumer Participation," *Journal of Health and Social Behavior* 14:368–374, December 1973.

[84] A.K. Tomeh: "Formal Voluntary Organizations: Participation, Correlates and Interrelationships," *Sociological Inquiry* 43:89–122, 1973.

[85] K.B. Partridge: "Community and Professional Participation in Decision-Making at a Health Center," *Health Services Reports* 88:527–534, June-July 1973.

[86] J.G. Cauffman et al., "A Study of Health Referral Patterns," *American Journal of Public Health* 64:331–356, April 1974.

[87] W.S. Blumenfeld and D.P. Crane: "Opinions of Training Effectiveness: How Good?" *Training and Development Journal* 27:42–51, December 1973.

[88] B. Gaoni: "Supervision from the point of View of the Supervisee," *American Journal of Psychotherapy* 28:108–114, January 1974.

[89] E. Viano: "The Styles of Management Inventory: A Methodological Analysis of a Training and Research Instrument," *Quality and Quantification* 7:91–106, 1973.

[90] C.J. Vander Kolk: "Comparison of Two Mental Health Counselor Training Programs," *Community Mental Health Journal* 9:260–269, Fall 1973.

[91] M.K. Goin: "Supervision Observed," *Journal of Nervous and Mental Diseases* 158:208–213, March 1974.

[92] P.S. Stephenson: Judging the Effectiveness of a Consultation Program to a Community Agency," *Community Mental Health Journal* 9:253–259, Fall 1973.

[93] D.M. Levine and A.J. Bonito: "Impact of Clinical Training on Attitudes of Medical Students: Self-Perpetuating Barrier to Change in the System," *British Journal of Medical Education* 8:13–16, March 1974.

[94] C. White: *Patient Characteristics and Supportive Behavior of Nursing Personnel in Nursing Homes,* Doctor of Public Health Dissertation, School of Hygiene and Public Health, Johns Hopkins University, Baltimore, 1973.

[95] T.S. Inui: *Effects of Post-Graduate Physician Education on the Management and Outcomes of Patients with Hypertension,* Master of Science Thesis, School of Hygiene and Public Health, Johns Hopkins University, Baltimore, 1973.

[96] R.L. Ebel: "Evaluation and Educational Objectives," *Journal of Educational Measurement* 10:273–279, Winter 1973.

[97] R.M. Balaban: "The Contribution of Participant Observation to the Study of Processes in Program Evaluation," *International Journal of Mental Health* 2:59–70, Summer 1973.

[98] K.W. Carlson: "Increasing Verbal Empathy as a Function of Feedback and Instruction," *Counselor Education and Supervision* 13:208, March 1974.

[99] C.M. Rossiter: "The Use of Videotape Recordings in Teaching Interpersonal Communications," *Speech Teacher* 23:59–60, January 1974.

[100] S.H. Surlin: "Broadcasters' Misperceptions of Black Community Needs," *Journal of Black Studies* 4:185–193, December 1973.

[101] L. Pankratz and D. Pankratz: "Nursing Autonomy and Patients' Rights: Development of a Nursing Attitude Scale," *Journal of Health and Social Behavior* 15:211–216, September 1974.

[102] L.A. Aday and R. Eichorn: *The Utilization of Health Services—Indices and Correlates: A Research Bibliography,* National Center for Health Services Research and Development, U.S. Department of Health, Education, and Welfare, DHEW Pub. No. (HSM) 73-3, 003, 1972.

[103] A. Antonovsky and H. Hartman: "Delay in the Detection of Cancer: A Review of the Literature," *Health Education Monographs* 2:98–128, Summer 1974.

[104] L.W. Green and B.J. Roberts: "The Research Literature on Why Women Delay in Seeking Medical Care for Breast Symptoms." *Health Education Monographs* 2:129–177, Summer 1974.

[105] E. Glogow: "Effects of Health Education Methods on Appointment Breaking. *Public Health Reports* 85:441–450, May 1970.

[106] M.R. Greenlick, D.K. Freeborn, T.J. Colombo, et al., "Comparing the Use of Medical Care Services by a Medically Indigent and a General Membership Population in a Comprehensive Prepaid Group Practice Program." *Medical Care* 10:187–200, May-June 1972.

[107] A.V. Hurtado, M.R. Greenlick, and T.J. Colombo: "Determinants of Medical Care Utilization: Failure to Keep Appointments," *Medical Care* 11:189–198, May-June 1973.

[108] O.C. Stine, C. Chuaqui, C. Jimenez, et al., "Broken Appointments at a Comprehensive Clinic for Children," *Medical Care* 6:332–339, July-August 1968.

[109] M.B. Sussman, E.K. Caplan, M.R. Haug, et al., *The Walking Patient: A Study in Outpatient Care,* Cleveland: The Press of Western Reserve University, 1967.

[110] J.F. Caldwell, S. Cobb, M.D. Dowling, et al., "The Dropout Problem in an Antihypertensive Treatment," *Journal of Chronic Diseases* 22:579–592, February 1970.

[111] F.A. Finnerty, Jr., E.C. Mattie, and F.A. Finnerty, III: "Hypertension in the Inner City. I Analysis of Clinic Dropouts," *Circulation* 47:73–75, January 1973.

[112] A.F. Williams and H. Wechsler: "Interrelationships of Preventive Actions in Health and Other Areas," *Health Services Reports* 87:969–976, December 1972.

[113] J. Steele and W.H. McBroom: "Conceptual and Empirical Dimensions of Health Behavior," *Journal of Health and Social Behavior* 13:382–392, December 1972.

[114] I.M. Rosenstock: "The Health Belief Model and Preventive Health Behavior," *Health Education Monographs* 2:354–386, Winter 1974.

[115] M.H. Becker: "The Health Belief Model and Sick Role Behavior," *Health Education Monographs* 2:409–419, Winter 1974.

[116] S.V. Kasl: "The Health Belief Model and Behavior Related to Chronic Illness," *Health Education Monographs* 2:433–454, Winter 1974.

[117] J.H. Mitchell: "Compliance with Medical Regimens: An Annotated Bibliography," *Health Education Monographs* 2:75–87, Spring 1974.

[118] L.W. Green: "Site- and Symptom-Related Factors in the Secondary Prevention of Cancer," in Bernard Fox (ed.), *Applying Behavioral Sciences to Cancer Control,* National Cancer Institute, Bethesda, in press.

[119] Nathan Maccoby: *Achieving Behavior Change Via Mass Media and Interpersonal Communication,* Paper presented at Symposium on Health Maintaining Behavior, January 30, 1975.

[120] "The Value of Cervical Cytology," *Lancet* 1236–1237, December 9, 1972.

[121] Keith J. Randall, "Cancer Screening by Cytology," *Lancet* 1303. November 30, 1974.

[122] Philip Strax, Louis Venet, and Sam Shapiro, "Value of Mammography in Reduction of Mortality from Breast Cancer in Mass Screening," *The American Journal of Roentgenology, Radium Therapy, and Nuclear Medicine* 3:686, 1973.

[123] Radical vs Simple vs. Simple with Radiation, NIH's National Surgical Adjuvant Breast Project headed by Dr. Bernard Fisher. University of Pittsburgh, Pennsylvania.

[124] National Center for Health Statistics: Chronic Conditions and Limitations of Activity and Mobility: United States, July 1965-June 1967. (Vital and Health Statistics, Public Health Service Publication No. 1000, Series 10, No. 61). Washington, D.C., National Center for Health Statistics, 1971.

[125] Commission on Chronic Illness. *Chronic Illness in the United States,* Vol. III, *Chronic Illness in a Rural Area.* Cambridge, Mass., Harvard University Press, 1959, page 578.

[126] Lawrence D. Haber, "Identifying the Disabled: Concepts and Methods in the Measurement of Disability," Report No. 1 of the Social Security Survey of the disabled, 1966. Social Security Administration, U.S. Department of Health, Education, and Welfare, Washington, D.C., 1967.

[127] Lawrence D. Haber and Richard T. Smith. "Disability and Deviance: Normative Adaptations of Role Behavior," *American Sociological Review,* 36:1, 1970.

[128] F.I. Mahoney and D.W. Barthel, "Functional Evaluation: The Barthel Index," *Md. State Med. J.* 14:61, 1965.

[129] M.W. Linn, "A Rapid Disability Rating Scale," *J. Am. Geriatr. Soc.* 15:211, 1967.

[130] S. Katz, A.B. Ford, R.W. Moskowitz, B.A. Jackson, and M.W. Jaffe, "Studies of Illness in the Aged: The Index of ADL, A Standardized Measure of Biological and Physiological Function," *JAMA* 185:914, 1963.

[131] S. Katz, Thomas D. Downs, Helen R. Cash, and Robert C. Grotz, "Progress in Development of the Index of ADL," *The Gerontologist* 10:1, Part 1, 1970.

[132] Jean Downes and Marguerite Keller. "The Risk of Disability for Persons With Chronic Disease," *The Milbank Memorial Fund Quarterly* 30:313–314, 1952.

[133] Commission on Chronic Illness, *Chronic Illness in the United States,* Vol. IV, *Chronic Illness in a Large City,* Cambridge, Mass. Harvard University, 1958, p. 375–377.

[134] *Illness and Health Care in Canada, Canadian Sickness Survey, 1950–51.* Published by the Queen's Printer and Controller of Stationery, Ottawa, Canada, 1960, p. 25.

[135] S. Katz, Amasa B. Ford, Thomas D. Downs, and Mary Adams. "Chronic Disease Classification in Evaluation of Medical Care Programs," *Medical Care* VII:2, 1969.

[136] S. Katz, Amasa B. Ford, Thomas D. Downs, Mary Adams, and Dorothy Rusby. *Effects of Continued Care: A Study of Chronic Illness In The Home,* Department of Health, Education, and Welfare Publication No. 73-3010, U.S. Department of Health, Education, and Welfare, Washington, D.C., 1972.

[137] Ellen W. Jones, *Patient Classification for Long-Term Care: User's Manual,* Department of Health, Education, and Welfare Publication No. HRA74-3107, U.S. Department of Health, Education, and Welfare, Washington, D.C., 1973.

[138] C. Amechi Akpom, S. Katz, and Paul M. Densen. "Methods of Classifying Disability and Severity of Illness in Ambulatory Care Patients," *Medical Care* 11:2, 1973.

[139] Clearinghouse on Health Indexes, Division of Analysis, National Center for Health Statistics: DHEW, Rockville, Maryland.

[140] Vital and Health Statistics, Data Evaluation and Methods Research, DHEW, NCHS: *An Index of Health: Mathematical Models,* Series 2, No. 5; *Conceptual Problems in Developing an Index to Health,* Series 2, No. 17; *Disability Components for an Index of Health,* Series 2, No. 42.

[141] Marsha Corey. "The State of Organized Family Planning Programs in the United States, 1973," *Family Planning Perspectives* 1:15, 1974.

[142] James A. Sweet. "Differentials in the Rate of Fertility Decline 1960–1970," *Family Planning Perspectives* 2:103, 1974.

[143] Caspar W. Weinberger. "Population and Family Planning," *Family Planning Perspectives* 3:171, 1974.

[144] Gerald Sparer, Louise Okada, and Stanley Tillinghast. "How Much Do Family Planning Programs Cost?," *Family Planning Perspectives*. 2:100, 1973.

[145] Gordon W. Perkins. "Measuring Clinic Performance," *Family Planning Perspectives* 1:37, 1969.

[146] Jean Hutchinson. "Using TV to Recruit Family Planning Patients," *Family Planning Perspectives* 2:8, 1970.

[147] Carl W. Taylor et al. "Assessment of a Family Planning Program: Contraceptive Services and Fertility in Atlanta, Georgia," *Family Planning Perspectives* 2:25, 1970.

[148] National Center for Health Statistics, *Decayed, Missing, and Filled Teeth Among Children*, Vital and Health Statistics, Series 11, No. 106. DHEW Pub. No. (HSM) 72-1003. Washington, U.S. Government Printing Office, Aug. 1972.

[149] National Center for Health Statistics, *Periodontal Disease and Oral Hygiene Among Children*, Vital and Health Statistics, Series 11, No. 117. DHEW Pub. No. (HSM) 72-1060. Washington, U.S. Government Printing Office, June 1972.

[150] H.K. Schonfeld. "Dental Evaluation Systems in the United States," *Public Health Reviews* 4:403, 1974.

[151] Helen M. Wallace, Hyman Goldstein, and Allan C. Oglesby. "The Health and Medical Care of Children under Title XIX Medicaid," *AJPH* 5:501, 1974.

[152] Ann-Marie Foltz. "The Development of Ambiguous Federal Policy: Early and Periodic Screening, Diagnosis and Treatment (EPSDT)," *The Milbank Memorial Fund Quarterly, Health and Society* 1:35, Winter, 1975.